Expert Decision Making on Opioid Treatment

Expert Decision Making on Opioid Treatment

Jane C. Ballantyne, MD, FRCA

Professor of Education and Research
Department of Anesthesiology and Pain Medicine
University of Washington School of Medicine
Seattle, Washington

David J. Tauben, MD

Clinical Associate Professor
Department of Medicine
Department of Anesthesia and Pain Medicine
University of Washington School of Medicine
Seattle, Washington

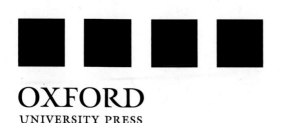

OXFORD
UNIVERSITY PRESS

OXFORD
UNIVERSITY PRESS

Oxford University Press is a department of the University of Oxford.
It furthers the University's objective of excellence in research, scholarship,
and education by publishing worldwide.

Oxford   New York
Auckland   Cape Town   Dar es Salaam   Hong Kong   Karachi
Kuala Lumpur   Madrid   Melbourne   Mexico City   Nairobi
New Delhi   Shanghai   Taipei   Toronto

With offices in
Argentina   Austria   Brazil   Chile   Czech Republic   France   Greece
Guatemala   Hungary   Italy   Japan   Poland   Portugal   Singapore
South Korea   Switzerland   Thailand   Turkey   Ukraine   Vietnam

Oxford is a registered trademark of Oxford University Press in the UK
and certain other countries.

Published in the United States of America by
Oxford University Press
198 Madison Avenue, New York, NY 10016

Library of Congress Cataloging-in-Publication Data
Expert decision making on opioid treatment/[edited by] Jane C. Ballantyne,
David J. Tauben.
   p. ; cm.—Includes bibliographical references and index.
   ISBN 978-0-19-976888-2 (alk. paper)
   I. Ballantyne, Jane C, – II. Tauben, David J.
   [DNLM: 1. Analgesics, Opioid—therapeutic use.   2. Chronic Pain—drug
   therapy.   3. Chronic Disease—drug therapy.   4. Diagnosis, Differential.
   5. Pain Management—methods. WL 704.6]
   LC Classification not assigned
   616'.0472—dc
   232012030810

9 8 7 6 5 4 3 2 1
Printed in the United States of America
on acid-free paper

Preface

Opioid treatment for chronic pain has been popularized over the past few decades, and opioid usage has increased severalfold. For example, in Britain, the prescribing of strong opioids in the community has risen by 70% since 2003, while in the United States, it has risen by 200% since 2000. Opioid treatment of chronic pain increased for several reasons: a sense that chronic pain had previously been undertreated; strong underwriting of medical education by drug companies anxious to sell new "designer" opioids; and lifting of the stigma associated with opioids, particularly as pain advocacy groups reestablished opioids as necessary and appropriate treatment for acute and cancer pain. What has emerged is that there are several limitations to chronic opioid treatment. First and foremost, efficacy is not always maintained during prolonged opioid treatment. While select patients seem to do well and experience good pain relief that improves their functioning and well-being, there are other patients who do not achieve such a good outcome. For these patients, over time, increasing doses provide a less useful effect, with failure to meet the treatment goal and, worse still, compromise due to the side effects and complications of high-dose opioid therapy. Complications include opioid refractoriness, or failure to obtain pain relief when needed for acute pain. Prescription opioid abuse has emerged as a significant problem and is now seen as a societal problem of enormous proportion in those countries where permissive use of opioids for pain has occurred.

What has become clear in this unfortunate history is that nonspecialists were persuaded to prescribe opioids before they could possibly understand the complexity of the treatment. So great were the pressures to prescribe—from drug companies, advocates, and many well-meaning people who saw opioids as the panacea for suffering—that opioids were prescribed indiscriminately. It became almost impossible to deny opioids without seeming inhumane. What we learned, though, is that while carefully selected and managed opioid therapy can benefit certain patients, casual use fails in several respects. What is needed, then, is a vast educational effort to help clinicians understand some of the complexities of opioid therapy, in particular, how to select patients and subsequently manage and monitor them so as to achieve continued efficacy without losing control of pain and drug use.

While no one educational effort can solve the problem, this book aims to provide clinicians with expert opinion on how to manage certain common scenarios involving opioid management of chronic pain. This is particularly important for primary care providers, who are most often challenged by the difficult decision making required to manage complex chronic pain. The book consists of 11 separate chapters, each prefaced by a clinical case that serves as the basis for discussion on how clinicians can incorporate a number of complex considerations in formulating a treatment plan that either includes or advisedly excludes opioids. The chapters are written by experts in the management of each diagnosis category, whose experience in treating the condition is applied to the role of opioids specifically. There are chapters on functional pain, chronic pediatric pain, chronic cancer pain, chronic painful disease, pain after trauma, pain with disability, and, finally, saying no to opioids. Authors are international and internationally recognized. While regulatory issues and drug availability differ from country to country, the principles of safe, effective, and humane drug choices apply across countries. It is these principles that are explored in this book. We hope that the book serves as a resource for anybody wanting to explore the role of opioids in the treatment of chronic pain under the capable guidance of international experts.

Jane Ballantyne and David Tauben

Contents

Contributors

Jane C. Ballantyne, MD, FRCA

Professor of Education and Research
Department of Anesthesiology and
Pain Medicine
University of Washington School
of Medicine
Seattle, WA

William C. Becker, MD

VA Connecticut Healthcare
System
Yale University
West Haven, CT

Shane Brogan, MB, BCh

Department of Anesthesiology
Huntsman Cancer Institute
Pain Management Center
University of Utah
Salt Lake City, UT

Stephen C. Brown, MD, FRCPC

Associate Professor
Department of Anesthesia
University of Toronto
Staff Anesthesiologist
Medical Director Chronic
Pain Clinic and Department of
Anesthesia and Pain Medicine
The Hospital for Sick Children
Toronto, Canada

Perry G. Fine, MD

Department of Anesthesiology
Huntsman Cancer Institute
Pain Management Center
University of Utah
Salt Lake City, UT

Lisa Isaac, MD, FRCP(C)

Staff in Anesthesiology and Pain
Medicine
Department of Anesthesia and
Pain Medicine
The Hospital for Sick Children
and
Assistant Professor, University of
Toronto
Toronto, Canada

Robert N. Jamison, PhD

Pain Management Center
Brigham and Women's Hospital
Harvard Medical School
Chestnut Hill, MA

Eija Kalso, MD, DMedSci

Pain Clinic
Helsinki University Central
Hospital
Helsinki, Finland

Robert D. Kerns, PhD

VA Connecticut Healthcare System
Yale University
West Haven, CT

Daniel Krashin, MD

Pain Fellow
Department of Anesthesiology and
Pain Medicine
University of Washington Medical
Center, Seattle, WA

Patricia A. McGrath, PhD

Scientific Director
Pain Innovations Inc.
Ontario, Canada

Edward Michna, MD, JD
Assistant Professor
Pain Management Center
Brigham and Women's Hospital
Harvard Medical School
Chestnut Hill, MA

James P. Robinson, MD, PhD
Professor of Anesthesia and
Psychiatry
Medicine Center for Pain Relief
University of Washington
Medical Center
Seattle, WA

Seddon R. Savage, MD, MS
Medical Director, Pain and
Addiction Treatment Program
Silver Hill Hospital
and
Director
Dartmouth Center on Addiction
Recovery and Education
Dartmouth Medical School
Hanover, NH

Juliana Serraillier, BS
Research Assistant
Pain Management Center
Brigham and Women's Hospital
Chestnut Hill, MA

Prof. Dr. Claudia Sommer
Neurologische Klinik
Universitätsklinikum Würzburg
Würzburg, Germany

Julie Franklin Sorensen, MD, MPH
Head of Pain Services, White River
Junction VAMC
White River Junction, VT
and
Assistant Professor
Dartmouth Medical School
Hanover, NH

Catherine F. Stannard, MB, ChB, FRCA, FFPMRCA
Consultant in Pain Medicine
Frenchay Hospital
Bristol, UK

David J. Tauben, MD
Clinical Associate Professor
Department of Medicine
Department of Anesthesia and
Pain Medicine
University of Washington School
of Medicine
Seattle, WA

Andrea M. Trescot, MD
Medical Director, Algone Pain
Center and
Fellowship Director
Trescot Fellowship Program
Wasilla, AK

Jennifer Tyrrell, RN, MN
Clinical Nurse Specialist
Department of Anesthesia and
Pain Medicine
The Hospital for Sick Children
Toronto, Ontario

Priv.-Doz Nurcan Üçeyler
Neurologische Klinik
Universitätsklinikum Würzburg
Würzburg, Germany

Chapter 1

Pain Without a Pathoanatomic Diagnosis

Catherine F. Stannard

The Case

Robert is a 52-year-old man who was referred to our pain clinic for rationalization of his opioid medication. He presented with abdominal pain of 6 years' duration.

Robert had an ileostomy for ulcerative colitis at the age of 19 but had ongoing intestinal problems so had a panproctocolectomy the following year. He had no abdominal pain for 26 years other than for a very short period in his mid-40s when he had a parastomal abscess needing incision and drainage.

His abdominal pain started spontaneously, and multiple gastroenterologic investigations failed to identify a cause for his symptoms. A histologic specimen from his original procedure confirmed the diagnosis of ulcerative colitis. Other diagnoses recorded in the notes included "functional pain," "nonorganic pain," "medically unexplained symptoms," and "pain of psychological origin." Because of his total colectomy, he met neither the Manning[1] nor the Rome II[2] criteria for irritable bowel syndrome. Urodynamic investigations and nerve conduction studies were normal.

He was referred to a pain team, who gave him a diagnosis of abdominal cutaneous nerve entrapment syndrome. Multiple local anesthetic procedures failed to provide any symptomatic relief. The patient moved to another city, where he was referred to a pain service that suggested further investigations, but the local gastrointestinal surgery team felt that his previous diagnostic tests were conclusive. The pain service carried out further ultrasound-guided nerve blocks in and around the pelvis, which did not provide pain relief. He was tried on a range of oral antineuropathic pain medications and even had trials of intravenous lidocaine and ketamine. He was given a trial of intrathecal opioid therapy that did not alter his pain, but one of the effects of the treatment was to provoke outbursts of angry behavior over which he felt he had no control, and he discharged himself from the hospital. He was referred to a pain psychologist.

When he presented to our service, he had pain arising in the lower abdomen radiating to the rectal stump. He described it as a burning sensation with vibration in the same territory and a sensation of something trying to punch its way out from the inside. Pain was unaffected by stoma function, eating, exercise, bladder function, or local pressure. His symptoms were present most of the time, but there were occasional days when he was symptom free. He found these remissions difficult to deal with as they imposed a regular cycle of raised expectations and dashed hopes.

Robert's medication included mirtazapine 45 mg daily in addition to morphine sustained release 400 mg bid and oral morphine liquid 240 mg tid. He frequently took supplementary doses of sustained-release morphine tablets in the middle of the day and also substantially self-escalated his liquid morphine dose. On his worst days the total morphine daily dose was estimated at 3000 mg. This pattern of overuse resulted in regular need for early prescription refills, which his general practitioner issued as the patient's pain was unremitting.

Robert was otherwise well. He had a history of depression 15 years previously at the time of being dismissed from his job. His mood improved quickly on this occasion with use of antidepressant medication. His mood worsened again with the onset of his pain, soon after which he lost his job as a sales manager. He felt that opioid therapy had caused a change in his personality and "caused his life to unravel." His relationship with his partner ended acrimoniously and he lost his house. He moved to live with his elderly mother and became profoundly depressed with frequent suicidal ideation, although the need to look after his mother prevented him from ending his life.

List of Considerations

1. Lack of diagnosis or explanation for pain
2. Progression to high dose with accompanying dysfunction
3. Methods for weaning

Considerations and Clinical Discussion

Diagnostic Challenges in Pain Medicine

A patient presenting with a symptom of pain without identifiable organic pathology may be described as having "medically unexplained symptoms" or "nonorganic symptoms." The patient may fulfill criteria for one of a number of defined disorders including factitious disorder, malingering (distinguished from factitious disorder on the basis of motivation, usually for financial or other gain), or somatoform disorder. These diagnoses, although rigorously defined, are the subject of some debate, and the final diagnosis may depend on the specialty, perceptions, and prejudices of the physician. For example, disorders such as chronic low back pain and complex regional pain syndromes may be classified as types of somatoform disorder as defined in the *Diagnostic and Statistical Manual of Mental Disorders,* 4th edition (DSM-IV),[3] whereas these would be considered discrete pathophysiologic entities by specialists in pain medicine. The term *functional pain syndrome* encompasses a number of poorly defined pain disorders including fibromyalgia syndrome, interstitial cystitis, and temporomandibular joint dysfunction. Again, attributing the term *functional* to these disorders is controversial as many such conditions are characterized by well-defined central and peripheral nervous system changes and adaptations. Functional pain syndromes are discussed in a separate chapter of this book, but currently the use of long-term opioids for pain relief in these circumstances is usually agreed to be inappropriate.[4]

The clinicians managing this case did not come to any agreement regarding diagnosis. His gastroenterologists decided he would have fulfilled the criteria for irritable bowel syndrome had he not had a colostomy; a surgeon described the patient as having "pain of psychological origin"; a diagnosis of "functional abdominal pain" was made when the patient was assessed by an insurance company in relation to his income protection policies; and two of his pain physicians commented that "visceral hyperalgesia" was contributory to his symptoms. The latter was important as the identification of a potential scientific explanation for his pain (albeit rather loose) may have influenced the willingness of his physicians to continue prescribing opioids.

Given the context of his referral to our pain service, it was important to ensure that the patient was not manufacturing symptoms for the purpose of misusing or diverting opioids. The patient had been observed taking high-dose morphine by hospital staff during his inpatient admission with no apparent additional effects compared to his presentation in the outpatient department (see below). The team agreed that the patient was using high-dose opioids in an attempt to control symptoms and that diversion was unlikely (routine urine testing is rarely carried out in the United Kingdom if patients do not have a history of illicit substance misuse). The sharp and sustained rise in prescription of strong opioids set against a backdrop of guidance advocating caution and restraint in the prescription of these drugs raises questions regarding the impact of such guidance.[5,6] Several studies have demonstrated that patient groups who may be at risk of running into problems are frequently being prescribed opioids and may not be monitored appropriately.[7–11] Strategies for implementation of guidance and evaluation of adherence vary. It is important that providers of opioid prescriptions have ready access to and an understanding of the rationale for prescribing. We felt misuse was unlikely for a number of reasons. The patient had no prior personal or family history of substance misuse and neither used alcohol nor smoked. He had been asking for some time for support in stopping his opioid medication (particularly when he understood the hazards of his current dose) as he had concluded that it was having little impact on his pain. Additionally, review of his medical records showed that the escalation of his opioid dose from his starting dose of codeine to his current morphine regimen had been incremental, with the significant dose increases occurring at times of report of intolerable pain or visits to new specialists who suggested dose escalation in the absence of any other diagnostically supported treatment strategy. During his several admissions to the hospital, he was consistent in his dose reports, supporting our impression that he was using medication himself rather than attempting to divert it.

Whenever considering long-term opioid therapy for pain, clinicians should also draw on the available evidence for efficacy in the pain to be treated. However, there is insufficient evidence from the published literature to conclude that opioids work any better in one particular chronic noncancer pain disorder compared to another, although clinical trials of opioid therapy mostly specify nociceptive or neuropathic pain.[12,13] There is little published evidence for the effectiveness of opioid therapy in poorly defined pain syndromes such as fibromyalgia.[14,15] Though the results of imaging investigations and other tests are important when making treatment decisions, magnetic resonance imaging (MRI) is neither specific nor sensitive enough to determine treatment in isolation.

Robert's case exemplifies the importance of comprehensive assessment by primary care providers and appropriate medical and behavioral medicine specialists to recognize medical, social, and emotional influences on the experience of pain.

Why Are Patients Prescribed High Doses of Opioids?: The "Opioid Journey"

Opioids were prescribed for Robert to relieve his pain. At its simplest, when on a very high dose of opioid therapy and there is no relief of symptoms, the treatment has failed, yet Robert's clinical scenario is common and cessation of opioid therapy is rarely considered. It is illuminating to review the clinical notes of these patients to find out when, why, and by whom opioids were first prescribed and to discover why dose escalation persists over time.

Robert's "opioid journey" is very typical. He was started on codeine by his general practitioner soon after presentation. His gastroenterologist commented, "I really am at a loss to know what is going on with this man but he is in severe pain so I have given him a supply of meperidine tablets." Two years later Robert was using markedly increased doses of meperidine in a haphazard way. His primary care physician changed him to oxycodone, which appeared apparently unchanged in his colostomy bag (although he may have absorbed active drug from the tablet) and the patient perceived no beneficial effect. Transdermal fentanyl was ineffective, so he was started on sustained-release morphine in a dose of 300 mg bid supplemented with oral morphine liquid 60 mg qid. He requested increasing supplies of morphine, which, at 400 mg bid, seemed to help for a while. However, this was associated with significant mood swings of concern to the patient and his family doctor, and the patient asked for help from pain specialists to come off his opioids. He attended a local secondary care pain service, which offered a number of interventional procedures in an attempt to provide pain relief without recourse to opioids. These were ineffective. Two years later he presented to our service, by which time his prescribed liquid morphine dose had increased to 720 mg/day in addition to his modified-release regimen. His actual opioid consumption was considerably in excess of that prescribed.

Medical case notes tell only part of the story in relation to opioid prescribing. The patient is a key player in therapeutic decision making.[16] When asked, Robert felt that his report of increasing pain and lack of response to his existing dose of morphine were the prompts to his primary care physician to increase his liquid morphine supply. He commented, "When you're in pain, you just want something to stop it." It is noteworthy that from the time of his doctor first expressing concerns about his opioid regimen, Robert became the patient of a multidisciplinary pain service. This may have, in some way, endorsed his ongoing prescription. He was given diagnoses of abdominal cutaneous nerve entrapment and subsequently of "visceral hyperalgesia." Again, the presence of a diagnosis from a specialist may have reassured his prescriber. We have recently reviewed the notes of all patients presenting to our service on high-dose opioids, and a theme to emerge from our review is that high-dose opioid therapy is common for patients with a history of previous surgery. We speculate that the fact of surgery somehow "legitimizes" the complaint of pain. A prospective cohort study of patients receiving opioids for low back pain suggested that duration of opioid therapy was greater for surgical compared to nonsurgical patients, although in the cohort studied, surgery did not influence dose escalation.[17]

There is a substantial literature relating to influences on prescribing behavior generally and prescribing of opioids in particular. The dilemmas facing a clinician when asked to prescribe opioids by a patient in pain were described well over a decade ago, with medical, emotional, intellectual, and logistic factors playing a role.[18] More recent studies of physicians in a variety of geographic settings demonstrate remarkably consistent findings over many years, with concerns about tolerance, dependence, and addiction, and beliefs regarding efficacy of opioids for long-term pain being important determinants of physicians' willingness to prescribe opioids.[19–21] Prescriber characteristics such as gender, time since qualification, and specialist training in pain need further exploration.[22,23]

Patient Perceptions of Opioid Treatment

An interesting but not surprising feature of this case is that the patient expressed a wish to stop his opioids 2 years before he was referred to be supported in this aim. After having stopped his opioids, he reflected on his opioid experience, commenting: "It makes you sluggish, it makes you more aggressive, more abrupt. I relied on Viagra to keep my relationship going. If I forgot to take a dose of MST [slow release morphine], horrendous withdrawal symptoms set in. You've seen the junkies on the television—shaking, sweating, agitated. Exactly the same."

Good practice suggests that patients are counseled about the potential adverse effects of opioids before starting treatment, but recent studies suggest that patients may have different problems and concerns, including psychosocial problems, that they attribute to opioid therapy.[24] Additionally, patients' attitudes and concerns about treatment are more predictive of nonadherence (including overuse) than intensity of symptoms or side effect burden.[25] Concerns about medications also correlate with emotional distress and disability, and this may add to the difficulties of living with unrelieved pain.[26]

Stopping High-Dose Opioid Therapy: Strategies for Detoxification

Robert was switched to methadone as a tool to bring about a safe and substantial reduction in opioid dose. Methadone has a number of pharmacologic properties, which both confer advantages in the management of persisting pain and necessitate caution when prescribing the drug. Methadone has a high affinity for both μ and δ opioid receptors in addition to activity at the N-methyl-D-aspartate receptor and monoaminergic effects.[27-29] Methadone has a large volume of distribution and is protein bound, and slow release from extravascular sites gives the drug its long and unpredictable half-life, which brings a significant associated risk of accumulation and delayed toxicity. It may take 5 days or more to achieve steady-state and maximal analgesia. The dose of methadone depends on the current dose of opioid prescribed, and careful adjustment and close observation are needed to determine dose requirements.

It is our current practice in the United Kingdom to admit patients to the hospital for conversion from high-dose strong opioids to methadone (the practice follows the experience of palliative care physicians in a hospice setting) to minimize the risk of adverse effects, particularly respiratory depression. This may not be an option for all patients, especially in the United States, for a variety of insurance and practice constraints. The inpatient setting is reassuring due to close monitoring for opioid withdrawal, increasing pain, and other opioid adverse effects. Compliance with therapy is also improved. The patients have contact with the pain team daily, who reinforce that the goal of the intervention is to reduce opioid load rather than to improve pain control.

A number of different strategies for establishing a hospitalized patient on methadone have been described. The authors use a modification of the regimen described by Morley and Makin, in which the previous opioid regimen is stopped completely and methadone prescribed 3hourly (in a dose calculated from the previous opioid load) for 5 days, after which the total daily methadone dose is given in two or three divided doses.[30] The patient can usually be discharged on day 6 and the dose and dose interval adjusted over the next few weeks. For patients who decline hospital admission or where this is not possible, outpatient conversion to methadone has been achieved successfully. Because conversion ratios between morphine (and other opioids) and methadone vary depending on the starting dose of (nonmethadone) opioid, it is difficult to be prescriptive regarding the rate at which methadone is introduced. For patients whose starting dose exceeds 500 mg morphine equivalent per day, it is the author's practice to effect the change in increments. The patient would be asked to substitute 50 mg morphine equivalent (from his or her total daily dose) with methadone 5 mg every 4 or 5 days, with weekly formal review and access to advice between reviews.

Buprenorphine is a partial μ opioid receptor agonist used increasingly for the treatment of opioid dependence in the United Kingdom and elsewhere, both as maintenance treatment and for detoxification. The drug may confer some advantages compared to methadone in this context. The doses of buprenorphine used for detoxification are much higher than preparations licensed for use in persistent pain, and collaborative management with addiction specialists is recommended, particularly as published detoxification protocols relate to the opioid-addicted patient. The adverse effects of buprenorphine are similar to those for methadone, but buprenorphine is described by patients as less sedating and "mind numbing" than methadone.[31,32] Buprenorphine has particular advantages over methadone for opioid detoxification because withdrawal symptoms are less prominent than with full opioid agonists.[33] The plan for opioid detoxification in an addiction setting for a patient established on methadone is to effect buprenorphine induction and then reduce the dose of buprenorphine every few days. The use of an α_2 agonist, such as clonidine or lofexidine, to attenuate the side effects of withdrawal is also recommended.[34] Preparedness of the patient for the withdrawal effects of detoxification is an important determinant of outcome and in the case described allowed a more rapid than usual detoxification.[35] There is no published literature on the use of buprenorphine in detoxification from opioids used to treat pain. In this circumstance a direct switch would usually be effected from the opioid being used to treat pain to buprenorphine. In the absence of available protocols, individual treatment plans need to be worked out between addiction medicine specialists and pain specialists.

Ethical Issues

The frequent positioning of opioids as a therapy of last resort brings some specific challenges regarding cessation of therapy. There is a commonly held perception among clinicians and patients alike that opioids cannot be stopped because no alternative therapy is available. Withdrawing analgesia leaves the clinician feeling powerless to help and the patient with a sense of having been abandoned to manage his or her pain unsupported. This represents a misinterpretation of the situation. Opioids are analgesics only if they achieve the aim of reducing pain intensity. If therapy does not achieve this simple goal, the balance of benefits and burdens tips wholly in an unfavorable direction. The advantages of stopping opioid therapy then become more obvious when viewed as an intervention to reduce harms of treatment. A patient who is freed from the side effects of opioids, particularly in relation to cognitive impairment, may feel better able to engage in and succeed in the use of more general pain management strategies. This is reflected in current research findings highlighting problems of long-term opioid therapy from patients' perspectives.[24]

Despite the important role of the patient in prescribing decisions, there are fewer studies in the published literature relating to the role of the patient, rather than the physician, in influencing the prescriber to issue an opioid prescription. Studies suggest that patient demographic features, particularly ethnicity, may influence the likelihood of receiving an opioid prescription, with the consistent finding that white patients are more likely to be treated with opioids.[36,37] One interesting study investigated patient race and verbal and nonverbal behavior on the decision to escalate opioid dose. For black patients physicians were more likely to escalate dose if patients exhibited challenging behaviors rather than nonchallenging behaviors, and the converse was true for white patients.[38] It is also well documented that neither pain severity nor observed pathology has much influence over prescribing, whereas behavioral manifestations of pain and reports of functional impairment are more likely to prompt the prescriber to issue opioids.[39] In general, patients who seem to demand medications influence their doctors to prescribe, and concerns regarding the effect of refusal to comply with a patient's prescription request on the doctor–patient relationship have also been described.[40,41]

Comprehensive Assessment

Comprehensive assessment of Robert will allow both the patient and clinician to define the most important areas of unmet need. A discussion of not only the characteristics of his pain but also physical and mental health comorbidities in addition to current domestic, vocational, and emotional concerns and how these and the pain interrelate helps define a management plan. With this full picture, the degree to which an isolated intervention to reduce pain intensity will improve Robert's quality of life is placed in a clearer perspective.

Discussion of Benefits and Burdens

Opioids have an unusual place in public perception as especially efficacious compared to other pain-relieving interventions. It is important to make patients aware that opioid medicines do not guarantee pain relief and, indeed, are poorly effective in a number of pain conditions, with modest attenuation of symptoms the best expected outcome. The importance of assessing pain relief in relation to improvement in function needs to be agreed upon with the patient and goals of therapy identified.

It is helpful for patients to know that side effects are the norm during opioid therapy and that persistent side effects are likely to limit utility of treatment unless pain relief and improvement in function are substantial.[42–44] Potential long-term harms in relation to endocrine and immune dysfunction should be discussed, as should the possibility of opioids worsening pain when used in high doses for long periods.[45–51] If the patient has a clear understanding that opioids might help but might also cause undesirable effects, this can usefully underpin a discussion about the importance of stopping opioids when the therapeutic outcome is poor.

Agreeing When to Stop

The discussion between prescriber and patient in relation to starting opioids should include a documented plan of when to stop treatment. Given the primary aims of reduction in pain and improvement in function, it is sensible to conclude that if neither of these criteria is fulfilled after two or three reasonable dose adjustments (supported by active management of side effects), the harms of opioid therapy are likely to outweigh the benefits and the treatment should be stopped.

Initial Recommendations

We discussed the potential harms of continuing high-dose opioid therapy. The patient wanted to reduce his opioid dose at the earliest opportunity, and he agreed to be admitted to the hospital for conversion of his opioid regimen to methadone as a first step. He understood that the purpose of this was to reduce his opioid dose and side effect burden and that his pain might be unchanged. He agreed that when his opioid dose had been reduced substantially, we would then decide whether opioids were going to play any role in his long-term management. His continuing low mood remained a cause for concern, and he was encouraged to retain regular contact with his psychologist.

On the first day of his admission to the hospital, morphine was stopped and he was prescribed methadone 30 mg three hourly upon request for treatment of pain. He was monitored daily with a subjective and objective opioid withdrawal tool and had no signs of opioid withdrawal and no increase in pain. In accordance with the opioid switching protocol used in palliative care, on day 5 of his admission his prescription was changed so that his total daily dose of methadone was administered in two doses. He was therefore prescribed methadone 80 mg bid and he was discharged on day 6. He was reviewed regularly over the next 4 weeks. His pain was unchanged but he continued to feel somewhat mentally clouded. We discussed treatment options, and he requested a change to sublingual buprenorphine in an attempt to improve clarity of thinking. He was readmitted to the hospital to make this switch. His methadone was stopped the day before admission, and he was observed for opioid withdrawal. By the end of the first day, he developed symptoms of withdrawal—yawning, lacrimation, shivering, and malaise—and was given buprenorphine 2 mg sublingually. He was prescribed lofexidine to attenuate symptoms of opioid withdrawal. During the next 24 hours he had two further doses of buprenorphine, after which he declined further opioid therapy and was discharged on day 5 opioid free.

In the weeks following opioid detoxification, we had agreed that monitoring of Robert's progress would be the responsibility of the pain team. In this way we could address any problems that needed to be resolved before handing his care back to his primary care physician. Robert's abdominal pain continued, but the focus of care was his continuing low mood, particularly during episodes of worse pain. Additional unmet and other emotional needs emerged; in particular, the impact of his stoma on his self-image and confidence had never been addressed. The patient was reviewed by the hospital stoma team, and his feelings about his stoma were discussed extensively with his psychologist. Robert addressed his feelings of desperation during pain flare-up, and his cognitive therapy focused on the way his beliefs and reasoning became skewed during these episodes.

Long-Term Treatment Plan

Robert's experience of opioid therapy, his perceptions about the role of opioids in his changed life circumstances, and his undoubted unpleasant experiences during detoxification resulted in him becoming very opioid averse. His providers discussed with him that his experiences were not the result of exposure to opioid medicines per se but rather related to the complex interaction of his experience of his pain, additional social and emotional stressors, and a failure of all concerned to act on the observation that opioids weren't helping him.

Robert, however, continued to have episodic abdominal pain. He became very low in mood during flare-ups and found life intolerable during episodes of worse pain. A year after stopping opioids, during an episode of severe pain, he discovered and used a remaining supply of immediate-release morphine; this had a partial pain-reducing effect. He asked for an immediate assessment with the pain service. The patient, the pain team, and his primary care physician discussed next best steps. The team made a decision to retry opioids under controlled circumstances. Because of the sudden onset of pain and its intermittent nature, we agreed that use of small doses of immediate-release morphine was appropriate. He was asked to keep a diary of his pain symptoms, his opioid use, and his response to therapy. A fixed monthly dose was agreed upon after reviewing his diary for 2 months. Robert's continuing experience of opioids was evaluated at the time of issuing each prescription.

The decision to return to opioid therapy in this case was carefully considered, and concerns and uncertainties were clearly documented. Continued demonstrable benefit from opioid treatment was agreed upon as the prerequisite for continued prescribing. We discussed again the absence of a diagnosis in Robert's case, and our pragmatic conclusion points out the difficult decision making in these circumstances and asks questions that remain unanswered but which should inform future research.

Question

If we are uncertain about the presence or absence of a diagnosis, can we deny opioids?

Answer

Maybe these patients should fall into the broader group of "at risk" patients who are managed by appropriate monitoring and support.

Summary Points

- The use of opioids to treat pain symptoms in the absence of a diagnosis is likely to be ineffective.
- When starting opioids a dose should be agreed upon, above which, if ineffective, opioids will be tapered and stopped.
- Iatrogenic addiction is difficult to treat and significantly complicates the management of pain, both of known and unknown etiology.

- A relationship of mutual trust and credibility in decision making underpins safe opioid treatment.
- Although the use of opioids in functional pain syndromes and other pains of uncertain etiology is not usually recommended, in reality many patients presenting with persistent symptoms of pain are difficult to fit into a precise diagnostic category. If factitious symptoms or diversion behavior can be ruled out, a very carefully controlled trial of opioids may be a pragmatic solution with the proviso that the drugs are stopped as above if ineffective.
- Opioid therapy should be monitored closely, particularly in relation to efficacy and harms of opioids.
- Patients may need substantial support if opioids are to be stopped, including opioid switching and tapering and active monitoring of opioid withdrawal.
- Cessation of high-dose opioid therapy is important for harm reduction and often is a starting point with regard to ongoing pain management.

References

1. Manning A, Thompson W, Heaton K, Morris A. Towards positive diagnosis of the irritable bowel *Br Med J*. 1978;2(6138):653–654.

2. Rome III diagnostic criteria for functional gastrointestinal disorders. http://www.romecriteria.org/criteria/

3. American Psychiatric Association. *Diagnostic and statistical manual of mental disorders*, 4th ed. (DSM-IV). Washington, DC: American Psychiatric Association; 1994.

4. Chou R, Fanciullo GJ, Fine PG, et al. American Pain Society-American Academy of Pain Medicine Opioids Guidelines Panel. Clinical guidelines for the use of chronic opioid therapy in chronic noncancer pain. *J Pain*. 2009;10(2):113–130.

5. NHS Information Centre. http://www.ic.nhs.uk/statistics-and-data-collections/primary-care/prescriptions

6. Boudreau D, Von Korff M, Rutter CM, et al. Trends in long-term opioid therapy for chronic non-cancer pain. *Pharmacoepidemiol Drug Saf*. 2009;18:1166–1175.

7. Sullivan MD, Edlund MJ, Fan M, et al. Risks for possible and probable opioid misuse among recipients of chronic opioid therapy in commercial and Medicaid insurance plans: the TROUP Study. *Pain*. 2010;150(2):332–339.

8. Morasco BJ, Duckart JP, Carr TP, et al. Clinical characteristics of veterans prescribed high doses of opioid medications for chronic non-cancer pain. *Pain*. 2010;151(3):625–632.

9. Edlund MJ, Martin BC, Devries A, et al. Trends in use of opioids for chronic non-cancer pain among individuals with mental health and substance use disorders: the TROUP study. *Clin J Pain*. 2010;26(1):1–8.

10. Braden JB, Sullivan MD, Ray GT, et al. Trends in long-term opioid therapy for non-cancer pain among persons with a history of depression. *Gen Hosp Psychiatry*. 2009;31(6):564–570.

11. Weisner CM, Campbell CI, Thomas G, et al. Trends in prescribed opioid therapy for non-cancer pain for individuals with prior substance use disorders *Pain*. 2009;145:287–293.

12. Kalso E, Edwards JE, Moore RA, et al. Opioids in chronic non-cancer pain: systematic review of efficacy and safety *Pain*. 2004;112:372–380.

13. Furlan A, Sandoval JA, Mailis-Gagnon A, Tunks E. Opioids for chronic non-cancer pain: a meta-analysis of effectiveness and side effects *CMAJ*. 2006;174(11):1589–1594.

14. Goldenberg DL, Burckhardt C, Crofford L. Management of fibromyalgia syndrome. *JAMA*. 2004;292:2388–2395.

15. Häuser W, Thieme K, Turk DC. Guidelines on the management of fibromyalgia syndrome—a systematic review. *Eur J Pain*. 2010;14(1):5–10.

16. Ballantyne JC, Fleisher LA. Ethical issues in opioid prescribing for chronic pain. *Pain*. 2010;148:365–367.

17. Cifuentes M, Webster B, Genevay S, Pransky G. The course of opioid prescribing for a new episode of disabling low back pain: opioid features and dose escalation *Pain*. 2010;151:22–29.

18. Bendtsen P, Hensing G, Ebeling C, Schedin A. What are the qualities of dilemmas experienced when prescribing opioids in general practice? *Pain*. 1999;82(1):89–96.

19. Potter M, Schafer S, Gonzalez-Mendez E, et al. Opioids for chronic nonmalignant pain. Attitudes and practices of primary care physicians in the UCSF/Stanford Collaborative Research Network. University of California, San Francisco. *J Fam Pract*. 2001;50(2):145–151.

20. Nwokeji ED, Rascati KL, Brown CM, Eisenberg A. Influences of attitudes on family physicians' willingness to prescribe long-acting opioid analgesics for patients with chronic nonmalignant pain. *Clin Ther*. 2007;29S:2589–2602.

21. Morley-Forster PK, Clark AJ, Speechley M, Moulin DE. Attitudes toward opioid use for chronic pain: a Canadian Physician Survey. *Pain Res Manag*. 2003;8(4);189–194.

22. Hutchinson K, Moreland AM, de C Williams AC, et al. Exploring beliefs and practice of opioid prescribing for persistent non-cancer pain by general practitioners. *Eur J Pain*. 2007;11:93–98.

23. McCracken L, Vellerman SC, Eccleston C. Patterns of prescription and concern about opioid analgesics for chronic non-malignant pain in general practice. *Prim Health Care Res Devel*. 2008;9:146–156.

24. Sullivan MD, Von Korff M, Banta-Green C, et al. Problems and concerns of patients receiving chronic opioid therapy for chronic non-cancer pain. *Pain*. 2010;149:345–353.

25. Rosser BA, McCracken LM, Velleman SC, et al. Concerns about medication and medication adherence in patients with chronic pain recruited from general practice. *Pain*. 2011;152(5):1201–1205.

26. McCracken LM, Hoskins J, Eccleston C. Concerns about medication and medication use in chronic pain. *J Pain*. 2006;7(10):726–734.

27. Ebert B, Andersen S, Krosgaard-Larsen P. Ketobemidone, methadone and pethidine are non-competitive N-methyl-D-aspartate (NMDA) antagonists in the rat cortex and spinal cord. *Neurosci Lett*. 1995;187:165–168.

28. Davis AM, Inturrisi CE. d-Methadone blocks morphine tolerance and N-methyl-D-aspartate-induced hyperalgesia. *J Pharmacol Exp Ther*. 1999;289:1048–1053.

29. Codd EE, Shank RP, Schupsky JJ, Raffa BB. Serotonin and norepinephrine uptake inhibiting activity of centrally acting analgesics. Structural determinants and role in antinociception. *J Pharmacol Exp Ther*. 1995;274:1263–1270.

30. Morley J, Makin M. The use of methadone in cancer pain poorly responsive to other opioids. *Pain Rev.* 1998;5:51–58.

31. Soyka M, Horak M, Dittert S, Kagerer S. Less driving impairment on buprenorphine than methadone in drug-dependent patients. *J Neuropsychiatry Clin Neurosci.* 2001;13:527–528.

32. Fischer G, Gombas W, Eder H, et al. Buprenorphine versus methadone maintenance for the treatment of opioid dependence. *Addiction* 1999;94:1337–1347.

33. Gowing L, Ali R, White JM. Buprenorphine for the management of opioid withdrawal. *Cochrane Database Syst Rev.* 2009;8(3):CD002025.

34. Glasper A, Reed LJ, de Wet CJ, et al. Induction of patients with moderately severe methadone dependence onto buprenorphine. *Addict Biol.* 2005;10(2):149–155.

35. Law FD, Myles JS, Daglish MRC, Nutt DJ. The clinical use of buprenorphine in opiate addiction: evidence and practice. *Acta Neuropsychiatrica.* 2004;16:246–274.

36. Moskowitz D, Thom DH, Guzman D, et al. Is primary care providers' trust in socially marginalized patients affected by race? *J Gen Intern Med.* 2011;8:846–851

37. Cintron A, Morrison RS. Pain and ethnicity in the United States; a systematic review. *J Palliat Med.* 2006;9(6):1454–1473.

38. Burgess DJ, Crowley-Matoka M, Phelan S, et al. Patient race and physicians' decisions to prescribe opioids for chronic low back pain. *Soc Sci Med.* 2008;67(11):1852–1860.

39. Turk DC, Okifuji A. What factors affect physicians' decisions to prescribe opioids for chronic noncancer pain patients? *Clin J Pain.* 1997;13(4):330–336.

40. Schwartz RK, Soumerai SB, Avorn J. Physician motivations for non-scientific drug prescribing. *Soc Sci Med.* 1989;28(6):577–582.

41. Weiss M, Fitzpatrick R. Challenges to medicine: the case of prescribing. *Sociol Health Illness.* 1997;19:297–327.

42. Moore RA, McQuay HJ. Prevalence of opioid adverse events in chronic nonmalignant pain: systematic review of randomised trials of oral opioids *Arthritis Res Ther.* 2005;7(5):R1046–R1051.

43. Chou R, Fanciullo GJ, Fine PG, et al. American Pain Society-American Academy of Pain Medicine Opioids Guidelines Panel. Clinical guidelines for the use of chronic opioid therapy in chronic noncancer pain. *J Pain.* 2009;10(2):113–130.

44. The British Pain Society 2010 Opioids for persistent pain: good practice. http://www.britishpainsociety.org/pub_professional.htm#opioids.

45. Merza Z. Chronic use of opioids and the endocrine system. *Horm Metab Res.* 2010;42.(9):621–626.

46. Katz N, Mazer NA. The impact of opioids on the endocrine system. *Clin J Pain.* 2009;25(2):170–175.

47. Odunayo A, Dodam JR, Kerl ME and DeClue AE Immunomodulatory effects of opioids. *J Vet Emerg Crit Care* (San Antonio). 2010;20(4):376–385.

48. Sacerdote P. Opioid-induced immunosuppression *Curr Opin Support Palliat Care.* 2008;2(1):14–18.

49. Fishbain DA, Cole B, Lewis JE, et al. Do opioids induce hyperalgesia in humans? An evidence-based structured review. *Pain Med.* 2009;10(5):829–839.

50. Mao J. Opioid-induced abnormal pain sensitivity: implications in clinical opioid therapy. *Pain.* 2002;100:213–217.

51. Angst MS, Clark JD. Opioid-induced hyperalgesia: a qualitative systematic review. *Anesthesiology.* 2006;104:570–587.

Chapter 2

Opioid Therapy of Chronic Pain in Persons With Known Substance Use Disorder

Julie Sorensen Franklin, Seddon R. Savage

The Case

Jay Russo, a 42-year-old Gulf War veteran, presents for initial evaluation for back and left lower extremity pain of 2 years' duration.

Jay Russo's pain problem began approximately 3 years ago when a coworker dropped one end of an "I" beam, resulting in a "pop" followed by severe back pain and later pain radiating down Mr. Russo's left buttock into his lateral thigh and across the top of his foot to his great toe. Due to radicular pain concordant with subsequent magnetic resonance imaging (MRI) findings, Mr. Russo underwent L5-S1 discectomy, and immediately afterward his left lower extremity pain and weakness resolved and back pain improved. Unfortunately, between 6 and 12 months after surgery, his back and leg pain returned. Repeat MRI at that time demonstrated scar around the left L5 nerve root on gadolinium-enhanced images.

Mr. Russo describes his current pain as ranging between 5 and 9 out of 10 in intensity with an average pain rating of 7. He would be satisfied with a pain level of ≤4 out of 10. The pain is constant and worse in his left leg than his back. It is "tingling and shooting" in nature, and he can identify no exacerbating or alleviating activities. He has no leg weakness or bowel or bladder dysfunction. He is currently taking oxycodone/APAP 15/500 one to two tablets 4 to 6 times daily for pain. He recently relocated to the area and is about to run out of his medication. He reports that oxycodone/APAP is "the only thing that helps." He notes that when he first started the medication, 15 tablets per month gave him adequate pain control, but now up to 12 tablets per day provide inadequate relief most days. His goals include pain relief and ability to "be a father to my kid." He has a sedentary lifestyle. The last time he tried to rake leaves he "paid for it for days."

He states that he has taken his last oxycodone/APAP this morning and needs a prescription today. Recent records from his previous physician are not available at the time of the appointment. He carries with him notes from about 1 year ago.

In addition to the oxycodone/APAP, he has tried a variety of other treatments for his pain. He has had epidural steroid injections, facet injections, medial branch blocks, trigger-point injections, physical therapy, and chiropractic manipulation without improvement in his pain. Medication trials have included nonsteroidal anti-inflammatory drugs (NSAIDs) (ibuprofen, meloxicam, naproxen), lidocaine patch, tramadol, propoxyphene/APAP, and acetaminophen with codeine, which were not at all helpful. Gabapentin reduced his shooting leg pain but had no effect on his severe back pain, so he stopped taking it. He has had no recent behavioral health or chemical dependency treatment despite both mental health and substance use risks.

Past medical history available and reported includes multiple fractures, including left femur from a motor vehicle accident (MVA), right fifth metacarpal from a bar fight, and multiple rib fractures from a skiing accident, and asthma requiring albuterol once or twice a month. He is overweight with borderline hypertension and not on medication for it.

Mental health/substance issues are significant. Mr. Russo describes anxiety since he returned home from the Gulf War and is receiving no current behavioral health treatment. He reports difficulty falling and staying asleep and sometimes awakens with sweats and palpitations. Alcoholism has been a problem for him. He has had in-patient detoxification and outpatient intensive treatment. He does not currently participate in a recovery program but reports no alcohol use in 5 years. He smokes one pack of cigarettes daily and has for 25 years. He has recreationally used marijuana and cocaine in the past. He recently used marijuana for pain at the suggestion of a friend and found it helpful.

Mr. Russo has been married for 18 years. He has children ages 10, 12, and 15 years old, all living at home. He previously worked in construction but is now out of work and applying for disability on the basis of his back problems. His wife is not present for his visit, but he states that she is "losing patience" with his chronic pain.

Mr. Russo believes his father "had drinking problems," but he was never treated, and he died 2 years ago of lung cancer at age 72 years. His mother is 69 years old in good health. Siblings are healthy.

Physical examination demonstrates a casually dressed and groomed, well-appearing man, with slightly elevated blood pressure and a body mass index (BMI) of 32. Mr. Russo's mood is anxious. His affect is constricted. Thought process is linear and goal directed. He makes fair eye contact with the interviewer. His gait is mildly asymmetric, with subtle favoring of the left leg. Hips are level. Spine appears normally aligned. He is unable to bend and touch his toes. He is unable to squat and stand without using his arms. The lumbar paraspinous muscles are diffusely tender bilaterally. He expresses increased pain with extension of the back. He has decreased sensation to pinprick on the left over the lateral leg and top of the foot. Patellar and Achilles reflexes are normal and symmetric. He has 4/5 strength on the left for dorsiflexion of the great toe. Strength is 5/5 in all other areas tested. Seated straight-leg raise is positive on the left at 30 degrees for leg and back pain.

MRI with and without gadolinium performed 13 months prior to this visit demonstrates enhancement around L5 consistent with postsurgical scarring. Facet arthropathy and disc degeneration are present at multiple levels.

List of Considerations

- What is the physiologic basis of the patient's chronic pain?
- What other factors contribute to his experience of chronic pain?
- What are the patient's modifiable contributors to chronic low back pain?
- Is further diagnostic testing warranted?
- What treatments are available to address each of the contributors to his chronic pain?
- Is it possible that his current treatment is contributing to his chronic pain? How?
- Is this patient a good candidate for chronic opioids? How should his immediate need for prescription refill be managed? What are the risks of withdrawal?
- If opioids are part of the treatment plan, how will treatment be monitored? What is the maximum daily dose of oxycodone for this patient? How can tolerance be managed?
- How important is his history of alcoholism in terms of the risks associated with chronic use of prescription opioids? Which features of his history are reassuring? Which are concerning?
- Are there other "red flags" for opioid abuse or misuse?

Clinical Discussion

This is a 42-year-old man with chronic pain maintained on opioids who presents requesting an opioid prescription immediately.

His pain complaints, history, and imaging studies are consistent with L5 radicular pain from nerve root entrapment. The differential diagnosis would also include radicular pain with a contribution from S1 and sciatic nerve compression from piriformis spasm/piriformis syndrome. Centralized L5 and/or S1 pain may also contribute to his current picture.[1] Muscle spasm likely contributes to his low back pain. Discogenic and/or facet-mediated low back pain may also contribute to the patient's symptoms.

Further workup of his problem could include imaging or electrodiagnostic testing. He does not endorse a recent change in pain symptoms, a sudden increase in pain, or a new area of pain. He denies worsening lower extremity weakness, any urinary retention, or urinary or fecal incontinence, which would indicate the need for urgent MRI of the lumbar spine. In this situation, the MRI performed just over 1 year ago is adequate to explain his current symptoms and does not need to be repeated. If there is significant concern for sciatic nerve compression, electromyelograms (EMGs) could be helpful in distinguishing radicular pain from peripheral nerve compression. EMGs are probably not necessary at this time.

This patient is a deconditioned, obese tobacco smoker. Obesity,[2] tobacco smoking,[3] and deconditioning[4] may all contribute to chronic pain, and all are potentially modifiable. The patient should be counseled to stop smoking and given resource materials/assistance as available. He may be referred for dietary counseling and an exercise program. Physical therapy may be helpful in suggesting ways to exercise without placing more strain on the back. Pool exercises are often good for patients with back problems. Strengthening core muscles can be helpful in managing chronic back pain. A good physical therapist can help the patient develop a home exercise program to address these issues. Physical therapy may also help reduce muscle spasm.

This patient's current medications may be contributing to his experience of pain. He has been maintained on higher-dose short-acting opioids only. Short-acting opioids may be associated with fluctuating blood levels and unstable pain control. Furthermore, this patient's dose of oxycodone could potentially cause opioid hyperalgesia[5] in some patients, possibly worsening rather than alleviating his chronic pain.

This patient complains not only of pain but also of poor function. He reports that pain prevents him from working or even "being a father" to his children. Many patients, especially patients with posttraumatic stress disorder (PTSD), suffer from fear/avoidance behaviors. Fear of injury or worsening pain may prevent patients from doing anything physical. Patients with chronic pain may benefit from a functional restoration approach to help them learn how to understand and manage the functional limitations imposed by chronic pain.[6]

Psychological and social stress also contribute to a patient's experience of pain. This patient's unemployment and related financial stress as well as the marital stress he alluded to may intensify his subjective appreciation of pain and interfere with his sleep. Better management of life's stress may help him to experience less intense chronic pain symptoms. Sleep hygiene and possibly a medication to help with sleep may also be useful as poor sleep may contribute to chronic pain. Mr. Russo, a Gulf War veteran, describes symptoms that may be attributable to PTSD and/or depression. If he is suffering from a major psychiatric illness, it is likely amplifying his pain symptoms and also increasing his risk of opioid misuse.[7] Psychological consultation should be obtained to address these issues.

Initial Recommendations

It is important to consider both short-term and long-term management of this patient's pain, including whether opioids should continue as a component of management. Mr. Russo states that he has run out of his opioids this morning. He has recently relocated to the area. He has come to his appointment expecting a refill on this first visit, putting pressure on the clinician to make urgent decisions with incomplete information. Recent records from his previous prescriber are not immediately available, but the records from up to 1 year ago do not show a history of problems such as inconsistent urine toxicologies, early refill requests, lost or stolen prescriptions, receiving opioid prescriptions from multiple providers, or rapid development of tolerance with escalation of opioid dose.

Providing a prescription for the patient in the absence of documentation of more recent visits to his prescriber, especially considering potential risk factors in his history, raises a number of very important concerns. The patient may in fact be using his opioids as prescribed for pain, albeit by his own report not achieving satisfactory relief. But he could also be out of medications early due to misuse or addiction and/or he might be seeking opioids for diversion. The decision about providing opioids at this visit must consider these possibilities, and effort should be made to obtain as much relevant information as possible to inform the decision.

The patient should sign a release to allow the provider to gather information from his previous prescriber. A phone call could satisfy any questions or concerns. Records can often be faxed quickly if his previous prescriber is not available to speak on the phone. The state prescription-monitoring program (PMP) should be consulted if available. If information from the previous prescriber's office or PMP data cannot be obtained, searching the patient's name online may provide some legal history; evidence of recent operating/driving under the influence citations can sometimes be found. Urine drug screening would also document use of medications and screen for use of illicit substances. Given the history provided, the specimen should be positive for oxycodone and/or oxymorphone, a metabolite of oxycodone. Other prescription opioids should be absent. The presence of illicit substances (likely here given his admission of recent marijuana use) should prompt further assessment. Physical examination can assess for signs or symptoms of intoxication, withdrawal, IV tracks, or stigmata of heavy alcohol or drug use.

The clinician could decline to prescribe medications for any new patient requesting immediate refills until more information is available, explain the potential for withdrawal and provide palliative medications to reduce withdrawal-related discomfort, and at the same time initiate nonopioid treatments for comfort. This would ensure that medication provided by the clinician will not be misused or end up in the street if the patient has misrepresented his reasons for seeking care. However, it will also result in significant discomfort for the physically dependent patient who has been taking 90 to 180 mg of oxycodone daily. He is likely to suffer withdrawal, including sweating, anxiety, and poor sleep, for a few days.[8] In addition, it risks having the patient not return and thus forfeit a potentially valuable therapeutic alliance, and it could end up with the patient borrowing or seeking street sources of medications, which may represent a serious risk. On the other hand, this urgent and unprepared visit for what should be a scheduled and long-expected visit raises legitimate concern.

An alternative option is to explain the clinical concerns and provide a small, short-term prescription of medication and see the patient back soon to plan more effective ongoing treatment as more information accrues. This would encourage the patient to engage in the clinical relationship and allow the clinician to further and more carefully assess and address his pain, substance use patterns, mental health issues, and other clinical issues. And it will prevent the patient who is actually using his medication from having withdrawal and increased pain.

Which of these options is best would depend on the clinician's considerations given the details of the clinical scenario. Simply renewing the patient's opioid for a whole month based on the history provided by the patient in not likely a prudent option in this context.

As important as how to manage this patient's short-term needs is how he can be managed long term. The foundation of effective chronic pain management is usually a multidimensional biopsychosocial approach that empowers the patient in optimum self-management of the pain and functional improvement. This often includes an ongoing physical conditioning program; cognitive behavioral approaches to pain control; treatment of co-occurring disorders such as anxiety, depression, or substance use disorder; and strategic use of interventionalist approaches and nonopioid medications as indicated, with implementation of comfort interventions such as heat, ice, transcutaneous electrical nerve stimulation (TENS), stretch, relaxation, and others. Because Mr. Russo is deconditioned, functionally disabled, and at risk for alcohol relapse as well as other substance-related problems, and reports anxiety and possible depression and PTSD, such a comprehensive approach is important.

As emphasized, Mr. Russo is likely to benefit from renewed attention to behavioral medicine intervention for his pain problem. Some other specific therapies may be helpful for him. Gabapentin helped Mr. Russo in the past; it could be restarted. Alternatively, another anticonvulsant such as pregabalin could be tried. Antidepressants may also be helpful in chronic neuropathic pain; a tricyclic or heterocyclic antidepressant could be started for this purpose. A sedating antidepressant taken before bedtime might help with the patient's poor sleep as well as his pain. An antispasmodic might be cautiously considered as treatment for his muscle spasm. A sleep aid could help with his poor sleep. Avoidance of potentially habituating sedative hypnotics is recommended in this patient because of his history of alcohol abuse and addiction. Physical modalities to improve this patient's pain have been discussed earlier. Interventional pain management may offer some benefit to this patient. A transforaminal epidural steroid injection or trial of a spinal cord stimulator could be considered.

Depending on the availability and response to such treatments, he may or may not also be a reasonable candidate for ongoing opioid therapy. A pathologic basis of pain is suggested by history, pain description, and examination. And he reports symptomatic and functional improvement on opioids and seems to be using them appropriately. However, there are concerns in this history that suggest a higher level of risk for opioid misuse, including a history of substance abuse, active tobacco use, unemployed status, male sex, a (probable) history of major psychiatric disorder, a history of illicit drug use, and current marijuana use.[7] A history of alcohol abuse is a risk factor for opioid abuse or misuse.[9] Mr. Russo is not actively participating in recovery. Many practitioners believe that his risk of problems is somewhat higher than if he were actively participating in recovery, although definitive evidence supporting this theory is lacking.[10] Active tobacco smoking status and history of recreational illicit drug use in the past are both associated with a greater likelihood of problems with prescription opioids.[9] Many clinicians believe that working-age patients who are not working also have a greater likelihood of misusing or abusing opioids, but this has not been consistently demonstrated in studies. Patients with a significant psychiatric history are at higher risk for problems with prescription opioids, especially if their psychiatric problems are untreated.[7] This patient endorses anxiety and symptoms consistent with PTSD. Referral to a psychiatric or psychology provider would likely be helpful both to help his psychiatric symptoms and to reduce his chance of having problems with his prescription opioids.

Long-Term Plan

Mr. Russo's chronic pain and associated symptoms will likely benefit from multidimensional care as discussed earlier. If continuation of opioids as a component of care is contemplated, he should be engaged with an addiction professional for assessment and recommendations for further treatment to support continued alcohol recovery and deter other substance misuse or addiction. It is also important to consider whether opioid misuse or addiction could be present and actually exacerbating his pain and distress. If opioid addiction is suspected or identified and opioids are considered necessary for pain control, it will be safest to provide these using an addiction treatment paradigm, either through a methadone maintenance program or buprenorphine treatment. While these paradigms may or may not provide ideal opioid pharmacotherapy of pain, they will usually provide some level analgesia and safety must be considered a priority.

If opioids are to be provided using a pain treatment paradigm, it is appropriate to consider whether long- or short-acting opioids are the best option for this patient. There is no compelling evidence in the pain literature that long-acting opioids offer clear advantages over short-acting opioids.[11] However, the addictions literature indicates that rapid onset of short-acting medications with continuously fluctuating blood levels provides both greater reward and greater stress associated with withdrawal than steady blood levels of opioids[12,13] and thus may both be a greater risk for patients with substance use disorders and provide less stable analgesia. On the other hand, a recent study suggested that patients who use time-contingent medications (most often long-acting medications) have more concerns about control of their medications than those using as needed (more often short-acting) medications.[14] In addition, patients who choose to can easily adulterate some long-acting formulations for purposes of abuse, resulting in higher risk. The use of tamper-resistant formulations may reduce these risks somewhat.[15] Because Mr. Russo is using opioids around the clock for pain, it is reasonable to consider longer-acting opioids on a trial basis if continued opioids are indicated, but the best option for the patient may need to be determined through trial and error with observation and revisions of the plan as indicated.

If this patient, who has multiple risk factors for opioid misuse, is treated with chronic opioid therapy, it is important to follow him closely.[16] An opioid prescribing agreement should be obtained. Ideally, the agreement should include informed consent about the risks and benefits of chronic opioid use including addiction, tolerance, accidental overdose, and endocrine dysfunction among others. An opioid prescribing agreement should outline mutually agreed upon goals of treatment as well as conditions under which opioids will be continued and discontinued. Many clinicians agree that urine toxicologies should be checked periodically to establish the presence of prescribed medication and absence of other opioids and controlled substances.[17] The patient should be seen and examined on a regular basis, no less than once a month at least initially, given his current multiple problems. His response to treatment should be tracked including his pain, level of function, psychological health, and substance recovery. If tolerance develops, Mr. Russo is likely to request an increased dose of his opioid. However, increased opioid dose is associated with an increased risk of adverse events, and he is already taking more than 100 mg/day morphine equivalent.[18] An opioid rotation could be considered as an alternative to dose escalation.

Ethical Issues

Untreated pain may cause suffering and loss of function in physical, psychological, and social domains. Addictive disorders may cause similar suffering and distress in these domains as well. Thus, the use of opioids in an individual with a history of addiction, in this case to alcohol in the past, and with current tobacco and marijuana use, who may be at risk for relapse to addiction to opioids requires a careful balancing act. Clinicians have an ethical obligation of *beneficence*, which would in this context require attempts to relieve pain. At the same time they are bound by the principle of *nonmaleficence*, to do no harm, in this case to avoid addiction or diversion of the drug.

The goal is to relieve pain-related suffering and increase function and quality of life while avoiding relapse to addiction in a person with identified risk factors for addiction. If medications and other clinical approaches without addiction potential are not effective in relieving pain, the clinician must consider the risks and benefits of implementation of opioids. The principle of *nonmaleficence* demands care in structuring and monitoring opioid therapy in this patient. The clinician might therefore consider providing opioids in smaller quantities at more frequent intervals, having more frequent visits for support and supervision, supplementing care with the support of an addictions professional, conducting more frequent toxicology screens, or providing other interventions aimed at reducing risk.

An additional ethical challenge in this and the many similar cases is the need to obtain informed consent for treatment with chronic opioid therapy. Qualities inherent in opioid medications, especially at higher doses, may affect decision-making. In addition, individuals with an addiction history may be influenced by cravings or other symptoms of addiction. The ethical principle of *autonomy* demands that patients be free to exercise their preferences and discretion in electing medical treatment. However, opioids may cause effects in some persons that attract their use for reasons other than pain relief, including reward or euphoria, mood modulation, sedation, and sleep induction, and some patients may become addicted to opioids and experience a compulsive desire to use them in response to craving. The inability of the user to recognize the addicted condition is a cardinal element of the addiction. Therefore, a person with co-occurring pain and addiction may be unable to thoughtfully consider the risks and benefits of opioids. He or she may be influenced by addiction or a compelling desire to manipulate affective states when providing consent for chronic opioid therapy. Furthermore, he or she may not be able to judge the efficacy of the medication in relieving pain independent of its other effects.

In this setting, it is important for the clinician not only to rely on subjective assessment of pain on the part of the patient but also to observe changes in function and quality of life. Significant others, as well as co-care providers, may provide valuable observations that help shape care for the benefit of the patient.

It is additionally important in this context to respect the principle of *justice*, which does not permit discrimination against a patient based on diagnosis or other factors, in this case a risk for addiction. This principle may be served by recognizing a shift in the risk–benefit balance for persons at risk for opioid misuse and providing special supports to avert negative consequences when opioids are used or making aggressive efforts to provide effective alternative treatments.

Summary Points

Multidimensional management of pain that respects the complex biopsychosocial nature of chronic pain and empowers the patient in self-care is the gold standard of chronic pain management and has special value in patients with co-occurring substance use disorders.

Use of opioids as a component of pain therapy in patients with a history of substance use disorder may sometimes be indicated, but this requires a careful assessment of the risks and benefits of opioids for the individual, weighed against the efficacy, risks, and benefits of alternative therapies.

Patients with a history of substance use disorder are likely at higher risk for opioid misuse or addiction, but these risks can often be effectively managed with a carefully structured and well-implemented plan of care that includes engagement of appropriate co-care providers with requisite psychiatric, addictions, or psychological expertise.

Routine use of urine toxicology testing may help detect drug abuse, misuse, and co-occurring addiction to other substances.

Routine use of an opioid prescribing agreement helps outline the risks, goals, and expectations around opioid therapy and ensures mutual understanding of the plan of care. It provides an important basis for continuing or discontinuing care.

If opioids prove critical for satisfactory control of chronic pain but cannot safely be used by the patient, engagement in methadone maintenance therapy or buprenorphine therapy of addiction may be the best option for the patient.

References

1. Rutkowski MD, Winkelstein BA, Hickey WF, Pahl JL, DeLeo JA. Lumbar nerve root injury induces central nervous system neuroimmune activation and neuroinflammation in the rat: relationship to painful radiculopathy. *Spine (Phila Pa 1976)*. 2002;27(15):1604–1613.

2. Wright LJ, Schur E, Noonan C, Ahumada S, Buchwald D, Afari N. Chronic pain, overweight, and obesity: findings from a community-based twin registry. *J Pain*. 2010;11(7):628–635.

3. Jakobsson U. Tobacco use in relation to chronic pain: results from a Swedish population survey. *Pain Med*. 2008;9(8):1091–1097.

4. Smeets RJ, Wade D, Hidding A, Van Leeuwen PJ, Vlaeyen JW, Knottnerus JA. The association of physical deconditioning and chronic low back pain: a hypothesis-oriented systematic review. *Disabil Rehabil*. 2006;28(11):673–693.

5. Hooten WM, Mantilla CB, Sandroni P, Townsend CO. Associations between heat pain perception and opioid dose among patients with chronic pain undergoing opioid tapering. *Pain Med*. 2010;11(11):1587–1598.

6. McCracken LM, Keogh E. Acceptance, mindfulness, and values-based action may counteract fear and avoidance of emotions in chronic pain: an analysis of anxiety sensitivity. *J Pain*. 2009;10(4):408–415.

7. Wasan AD, Butler SF, Budman SH, Benoit C, Fernandez K, Jamison RN. Psychiatric history and psychologic adjustment as risk factors for aberrant drug-related behavior among patients with chronic pain. *Clin J Pain*. 2007;23(4):307–315.

8. Cowan DT, Wilson-Barnett J, Griffiths P, Vaughan DJ, Gondhia A, Allan LG. A randomized, double-blind, placebo-controlled, cross-over pilot study to assess the effects of long-term opioid drug consumption and subsequent abstinence in chronic noncancer pain patients receiving controlled-release morphine. *Pain Med*. 2005;6(2):113–121.

9. Ives TJ, Chelminski PR, Hammett-Stabler CA, et al. Predictors of opioid misuse in patients with chronic pain: a prospective cohort study. *BMC Health Serv Res*. 2006;6:46.

10. Ferri MAL, Davoli M. Alcoholic Anonymous and other 12-step programmes for alcohol dependence. *Cochrane Database Syst Rev*. 2006;(3):CD005032…

11. Chou R, Clark E, Helfand M. Comparative efficacy and safety of long-acting oral opioids for chronic non-cancer pain: a systematic review. *J Pain Symptom Manage*. 2003;26(5):1026–1048.

12. Marsch LA, Bickel WK, Badger GJ, et al. Effects of infusion rate of intravenously administered morphine on physiological, psychomotor, and self-reported measures in humans. *J Pharmacol Exp Ther*. 2001;299(3):1056–1065.

13. Butler SF, Benoit C, Budman SH, et al. Development and validation of an Opioid Attractiveness Scale: a novel measure of the attractiveness of opioid products to potential abusers. *Harm Reduct J*. 2006;3:5.

14. Von Korff M, Merrill JO, Rutter CM, Sullivan M, Campbell CI, Weisner C. Time-scheduled vs. pain-contingent opioid dosing in chronic opioid therapy. *Pain*. 2011;152(6):1256–1262.

15. Raffa RB, Pergolizzi JV Jr. Opioid formulations designed to resist/deter abuse. *Drugs.* 2010;70(13):1657–1675.

16. Chou R, Fanciullo GJ, Fine PG, et al. Clinical guidelines for the use of chronic opioid therapy in chronic noncancer pain. *J Pain.* 2009;10(2):113–130.

17. Interagency guideline on opioid dosing for chronic non-cancer pain: an educational aid to improve care and safety with opioid therapy. http://www.guideline.gov/content.aspx?id=23792&search=opioid. Accessed April 1, 2012.

18. Bohnert AS, Valenstein M, Bair MJ, et al. Association between opioid prescribing patterns and opioid overdose-related deaths. *JAMA.* 2011;305(13):1315–1321.

Chapter 3

Screening before Embarking

How to Screen for Addiction Risk in Opioid Prescribing

Robert N. Jamison, Juliana Serraillier, Edward Michna

The Case

Michael Smith is a 39-year-old disabled carpenter with a 6-year history of chronic back and right lower extremity pain. He initially injured his back from a fall at work. He was evaluated and treated by a number of health care providers and received physical therapy, many medications, and nerve blocks. He eventually had back surgery, which was complicated by a wound infection that ultimately led to a succession of four back surgeries with implantation and later removal of hardware. He is no longer considered a candidate for surgery. He reports that his back and leg pain have worsened since his first surgery. His primary care physician had been prescribing opioids for his pain but has relocated to another practice, and no other local providers are willing to prescribe opioids to treat his pain; he is angry that his health providers have abandoned him. He states, "I know that I will always have some pain, but I need help so that I can have a life."

At the time of his initial evaluation he described his pain as varying between 7 and 10 on a 0–10 scale. The pain was aching, burning, sharp, and pulling in nature, worsening with walking, lifting, bending, standing, or sitting for long periods. He had significant sleep disturbances and felt fatigued. He had problems with memory and concentration and felt isolated due to his pain. He reported a history of depression, current trouble with irritability, and often becoming agitated when around others. He stated, "I don't feel like a person." He denied any active suicidal ideation. He had been periodically meeting with a psychiatrist.

Mr. Smith described his childhood as difficult. He was 3 years old when his mother died in a motor vehicle accident and was raised by his aunt and uncle, who were abusive and not good caretakers. As a young adult he had been incarcerated for disorderly conduct while intoxicated. At the time of his first appointment he was married to his second wife and he had an 18-year-old daughter who lived with his ex-wife.

Mr. Smith smokes half a pack of cigarettes a day. He had a history of drinking alcohol daily but reportedly has been sober for the past 4 years. He describes prior abuse of multiple substances including cocaine. He has attended Alcoholics Anonymous and Narcotics Anonymous meetings and reported no use of "street drugs" over the last 10 years. He also had a history of hospitalization after accidently overdosing on prescription medication.

Other medical comorbidities include a history of pneumonia, osteomyelitis, asthma, and hypertension. His current medications include morphine sulfate, oxycodone, diazepam, citalopram, inhalers, and antihypertensives. He is hoping that opioids will continue to be prescribed for his pain.

List of Considerations

Medical comorbidities:
1. Failed back surgery
2. History of pneumonia
3. Osteomyelitis
4. Asthma
5. Hypertension

Psychiatric comorbidities:
1. Anxiety
2. Depression
3. Agitation and extreme irritability
4. Dysfunctional family background

Substance abuse history:
1. Alcohol dependence
2. Cigarette smoking
3. History of illicit substance use
4. History of accidental overdose

Clinical Discussion

Medical Comorbidities

Many people with complex pain such as Mr Smith's present with medical comorbidities. Medical disorders frequently increase impairment and disability, complicate and often interfere with successful pain treatment, and contribute to an increase in patient-reported pain intensity. In this case, as in many others, individuals suffering from chronic pain share a chaotic life history of unhealthy behaviors including tobacco use, alcoholism, and substance abuse. When disabled, many experience weight gain and further deconditioning. Chronic medical diseases also may require medications prescribed by multiple other providers, which include blood pressure and heart disease medications, inhaled bronchodilators, and sometimes blood thinners; drug–drug interactions can thus complicate treatment choices, and coordination among prescribers is of critical importance to avoid dangerous coprescribing. Chronic pain patients may report interactions among medications as "allergies." They may also have electronic medical devices implanted, such as pacemakers, intrathecal pumps, and spinal cord stimulators, complicating magnetic resonance imaging (MRI) evaluations that may be needed for thorough assessment and management. It is essential for prescribing clinicians to accurately identify past medical conditions and to communicate with all current treatment providers to avoid complications arising from uncoordinated medical care.

Psychiatric Comorbidities

Studies suggest that most patients with chronic pain present with some psychiatric symptoms. Many chronic pain patients report feelings of depression, anxiety, and irritability and have a history of physical or sexual abuse or a history of a mood disorder.[1,2] Close to 50% of patients with chronic pain have a comorbid psychiatric condition, and 35% of patients with chronic back and neck pain have a comorbid depression or anxiety disorder.[3–5] In surveys of chronic pain clinic populations, between 50% and 70% of patients with chronic pain indicate signs of psychopathology, making this the most prevalent comorbidity in these patients.[6–9]

Arkinstall and colleagues found a 50% prevalence of mood disorder in patients who were prescribed opioids, suggesting this to be a common diagnosis for chronic pain patients.[10] Another study found that physicians are more likely to prescribe opioids for non-cancer-related pain on the basis of increased affective distress and pain behavior, rather than the patient's pain severity or objective physical pathology.[11] It has been found that patients who have chronic pain with psychopathology are more likely to report greater pain intensity, more pain-related disability, and a larger affective component to their pain than those who do not have evidence of psychopathology.[12]

Patients with chronic pain and psychopathology, especially those with chronic low back pain, also typically have poorer pain and disability outcomes from treatments.[13–16] Studies have found a significantly worse return-to-work rate 1 year after injury among patients with both chronic pain and anxiety and/or depression compared with those without any psychopathology.[17,18] Patients who had chronic pain with low psychopathology had a 40% greater reduction in pain with IV morphine than those in a high-psychopathology group.[19] It is apparent that patients with a high degree of negative affect benefit less when trying to control their pain with opioids.

Many patients with affective disorders also have substance use disorders. Attempting to manage a comorbid affective disorder may result in decreased substance abuse behaviors, although patients may be at risk of relapse.[20–23] Hasin and colleagues found some patients abusing their pain medication as a way to alleviate their psychiatric symptoms.[24] This finding and other reviews suggest that individuals with a mood disorder who self-medicate for negative affect are at increased risk for substance abuse.[25] Because many patients with chronic pain frequently report mood swings and prominent anxiety and depression symptoms, it remains important to carefully monitor all patients for psychiatric comorbidity. This way, individuals self-medicating their mood fluctuations with analgesics will have a greater chance of receiving appropriate antidepressant and behavioral treatments instead of ineffective and potentially dangerous opioid analgesics.

Substance Abuse Risk and the Role of Screening

The pain literature indicates that physicians are able to better provide suitable treatment and care to patients with chronic pain once substance misuse causes are recognized.[26] For clarity of terms, *substance misuse* is the use of any drug in a manner other than how it is indicated or prescribed, whereas *substance abuse* is defined as the use of any substance when such use is unlawful or when such use is detrimental to the user or others.[27] *Addiction* is a behavioral pattern of substance abuse characterized by overwhelming involvement with the use of a drug. Addiction is generally understood to be a chronic condition from which recovery is possible; however, the underlying neurobiologic dysfunction, once manifested, is believed to persist.[28,29] Addiction focuses on compulsive use of the drug that results in physical, psychological, and social harm to the user. An individual who has an addiction to a drug continues to use it, despite harm. *Physical dependence* is a common phenomenon of all mammals taking opioids characterized by physical withdrawal symptoms when an opioid is discontinued. *Tolerance* is also a commonly observed phenomenon when taking opioids over time in which the individual becomes used to the drug and has a need for increasing doses to maintain the same effect. Both physical dependence and tolerance are typically found among patients who use opioids for chronic pain and are often unrelated to true addiction. Finally, *aberrant drug-related behavior* is behavior suggestive of a substance abuse and/or addiction disorder. Examples are selling prescription drugs, forging prescriptions, stealing or "borrowing" drugs from others, injecting oral formulations, obtaining prescription drugs from nonmedical sources, having multiple episodes of prescription "loss," repeatedly seeking prescriptions from other clinicians, displaying evidence of deterioration in function (work, home, family), and repeatedly resisting changes to therapy despite evidence of physical and psychological problems.

Misuse behaviors of prescribed opioid medication are determined by assessment and treatment protocols. These protocols help to identify patients who show signs of opioid misuse, because they provide the clinician with an overview of the patient's background and behavior. The US Department of Justice recommended efforts to improve identification of abuse and diversion of controlled substances by health care providers.[30] Physicians continue to struggle with providing the appropriate pain relief for patients while minimizing the misuse of opioid analgesics.[31]

Some patients may become psychologically dependent after long-term opioid use.[32,33] Other patients who are chronically maintained on high doses of opioids manifest impaired cognition, problems with psychomotor performance, and opioid-induced hyperalgesia.[34] Studies also suggest that a relationship exists between early misuse of opioids and addiction.[25] This relationship emphasizes the need for early detection of risk, close monitoring, and direct interventions when needed.

Patients who are typically at a lower risk for misusing opioids include those who are older; are generally compliant; have a record of rarely misusing any medication; show stable mood; are rational, thoughtful, and responsible; and generally have an easy-going personality. Risk factors for opioid misuse include (1) family or personal history of substance abuse; (2) young age; (3) history of criminal activity and/or legal problems (e.g., charged with driving under the influence [DUI]); (4) frequent contact with high-risk individuals or environments; (5) history of problems with employers, family, and friends; (6) history of risk-taking/thrill-seeking behavior; (7) smoking cigarettes; (8) history of severe depression or anxiety; (9) multiple psychosocial stressors; (10) history of childhood abuse; and (11) previous drug and/or alcohol rehabilitation.[35,36] Patients prescribed opioids should be monitored regularly and should be examined for experiencing any adverse effects. Appropriate follow-up care should include repeated psychological evaluations.

Screening Tools

There are a variety of assessment measures that can be used to help identify those patients who are prone to misuse their pain medications.[37] Structured interview measures have been published for assessment of alcoholism and drug use disorder based on *Diagnostic and Statistical Manual of Mental Disorders,* fourth edition (DSM-IV) criteria [38], but these measures have not been validated in individuals with chronic pain. Some substance abuse measures, including the CAGE Questionnaire, Michigan Alcoholism Screening Test, and Self-Administered Alcoholism Screening Test, were initially designed for other patient populations.[39–41] Using traditional substance abuse assessment tools may be beneficial for patients with a severe substance use disorder; however, these assessments may not be useful for individuals with chronic pain because there is a greater chance of a false positive with these measures. In general, there is a risk that a medication use disorder using traditional substance use disorder measures will be identified based on reports of tolerance and withdrawal when no disorder exists.

The Screener and Opioid Assessment for Patients with Pain—Revised (SOAPP-R) is a 24-item self-administered screening tool developed and validated for those persons with chronic pain who are being considered for long-term opioid therapy. The SOAPP-R is designed to predict aberrant medication-related behaviors.[42,43] This questionnaire includes subtle items that encourage the patient to admit to certain factors that are positively correlated with opioid misuse yet outwardly are not perceived to lead to reprisals. Any individual who scores more than an 18 on the SOAPP-R is rated as being at risk for opioid misuse. This screening tool has been found to identify 90% of those chronic pain patients who will eventually misuse opioids. It has been cross-validated in over 600 patients across the United States. The reliability and predictive validity of the SOAPP-R were found to be highly significant. Results of a cross-validation suggest that the psychometric parameters of the SOAPP-R are not based solely on the unique characteristics of the initial validation sample.[44]

The Current Opioid Misuse Measure (COMM) is a 17-item questionnaire developed and validated for patients who have already been prescribed opioids for chronic pain.[45] Several measures predict misuse behaviors in patients before they are prescribed opioids; however, the COMM helps to identify those patients who are currently misusing their prescribed opioid medication. The COMM was created to repeatedly document opioid compliance and improve clinician sense of appropriateness of opioid therapy. The COMM has been determined to be a brief but useful self-report measure of current aberrant drug-related behavior. The reliability and predictive validity in this cross-validation were found to be highly significant. Results of a cross-validation suggest that the psychometric parameters of the COMM are not based solely on unique characteristics of the initial validation sample.[46] Both the SOAPP-R and COMM include subtle items that are correlated with opioid misuse and are items patients tend to answer honestly.

Other validated measures have also been developed to screen patients with pain for addiction risk potential. The 5-item Opioid Risk Tool (ORT) is a validated brief checklist completed by the clinician that helps to predict which patients will display aberrant drug-related behaviors.[41,47] Scores of 8 or higher suggest high risk for opioid medication use disorder.

An additional rating tool, the DIRE (standing for diagnosis, intractability, risk, and efficacy), is a clinician rating scale used to predict suitability for long-term opioid treatment for noncancer pain.[48] It also attempts to identify beneficial factors of opioid use. Scores higher than 14 on the DIRE suggest a greater suitability of opioid therapy for pain patients.

The Pain Assessment and Documentation Tool (PADT) is yet another scale completed by the clinician; it provides a detailed documentation of the patient's progress, which also helps to objectively record a patient's care.[47,49] The Screening Instrument for Substance Abuse Potential (SISAP) is a self-report screening questionnaire for substance abuse potential based mostly on the alcohol literature.[50] Unfortunately, this and other similar measures lack cross-validation studies. When using any tools to assess risk of opioid misuse, it is important to consider the scores in context with patient background information and to take all information into consideration when developing a treatment plan.

It is important to note that scores of any clinical assessment tool used to determine abuse risk are not necessarily reason to deny opioids, but rather provide an estimate of the level of appropriate monitoring for the patient. Thus, although these clinical assessments are useful to estimate risk of noncompliant opioid use, the results are most useful to help determine how closely to monitor patients during opioid therapy.

What measures would be best to use? The SOAPP-R is a 24-item self-administered measure that has been cross-validated and would be recommended in routine practice to assess risk potential. Some prefer to use the

Table 3.1 List of Opioid Risk Screening Tools

- Screener and Opioid Assessment for Patients in Pain-Revised (SOAPP-R)
- Current Opioid Misuse Measure (COMM)
- Opioid Risk Tool (ORT)
- Diagnosis, Intractability, Risk, and Efficacy (DIRE)
- Screening Instrument for Substance Abuse Potential (SISAP)
- Pain Assessment and Documentation Tool (PADT)

5-item ORT as an initial screening tool because it is brief and easy to administer, but a limitation of this checklist is that it requires that the clinician be familiar with the patient. The 17-item COMM and PADT are used to assess follow-up measures of risk, and the COMM has the most validity. A benefit of the DIRE is that it gives information about suitability of opioids as well as assesses risk. Unfortunately, the ORT, PADT, DIRE, and SISAP mentioned previously have not been cross-validated; however, they may still be useful in clinical practice. Table 3.1 presents a list of these frequently used tools.

Urine Toxicology Screens

In the pain clinic setting, and ideally in treatment centers in general, a urine toxicology screen should be obtained at some point, especially when the transition from acute to chronic opioid use is established (e.g., after 90 days of continuous use). This screen can be compared with the patient's self-reported recent medication intake to identify the presence of any unexpected drugs (e.g., THC) or absence of an intended one (e.g., prescribed oxycodone).

Clinicians use urine drug screens to closely monitor patients' adherence to their prescribed opioid medication. Highly sensitive and specific urine screens (e.g., gas chromatography/mass spectrometry—GC/MS) help to identify the presence and quantities of prescription medications, presence of illegal substances, and/or absence of prescribed medications. It is important to know the cutoff levels used by the laboratory to determine the presence or absence of a drug. Also, certain drugs metabolize rapidly (e.g., alcohol within 24 hours) and other substances can be detected in the urine for an extended period of time (e.g., marijuana may be detected 2 weeks after use). Knowledge that certain drugs metabolize into other substances (e.g., hydrocodone into hydromorphone) will prevent accusations of misuse based on false-positive results. Even though the majority of patients prescribed opioids do not misuse their medication, it still is reasonable and important to document compliance for all patients on chronic opioid therapy by obtaining a urine screen at least yearly.

The combination of urine screens, self-report questionnaires, and behavioral observation methods has aided providers in properly identifying which patients are misusing their prescribed opioids. One study gathered urine toxicology results among 122 patients who were prescribed opioids for pain and found abnormal results in 43% of this sample.[51] Another study found 21% of the study patients with no obvious behavioral issues to have either a positive urine screen result for an illicit drug or a nonprescribed controlled medication in their urine. These results imply that some risk factors for opioid misuse may not always properly identify patients who do misuse their pain medication. An additional study of 226 patients with chronic pain surprisingly found 46.5% of the sample to have abnormal urine toxicology screen results.[52] In a retrospective study of 470 patients, 4 of 10 patients prescribed opioids also had abnormal urine toxicology screens.[53] These studies underscore the importance of urine toxicology screens along with behavioral observation and self-report measures to help identify aberrant drug-related behavior. Although immunoassay urine screens are often used as the first line of analysis, GC/MS urine screens provide useful results in being able to quantify the extent of illicit and prescription drug use. This type of urine toxicology screen is also able to detect drug metabolites, as well as determine whether the patient has attempted to adulterate the urine sample.[54]

Increasingly, patients with chronic pain are using marijuana for the treatment of their symptoms, and evidence of THC in the urine has become more prevalent.[55] There exists a great deal of controversy over the use of medical marijuana, specifically its use among pain patients prescribed opioids for pain.[56] Some clinicians feel that in order to be prescribed opioids there needs to be a record of clean urines. These clinicians also believe that use of marijuana is unacceptable when taking prescription opioids because of its association with abuse of other illicit substances. Other physicians feel that use of marijuana is not grounds for discontinuation of opioid therapy, although legal implications need to be considered. Nonetheless, the use of regular urine toxicology screens is important in identifying opioid misuse, and doctor–patient discussions about the responsible use of opioids are essential.

The Role of Screening

A randomized trial of patients prescribed opioids for noncancer back pain who showed risk potential for or demonstration of opioid misuse was conducted to see if close monitoring along with cognitive behavioral substance misuse counseling could increase overall compliance with opioids.[57] Patients identified as high and low risk for misuse of opioids were followed for 6 months and completed prestudy and poststudy questionnaires as well as monthly electronic diaries. Overall, this study demonstrated a positive effect of improving opioid compliance, particularly among those patients at high risk for misuse of opioids. The results of this study suggested that compliance training along with very careful monitoring of high-risk patients for opioid misuse can be incorporated as part of a multidisciplinary pain program. This program was shown to help improve compliance with opioids and reduce the number of individuals who are discharged from treatment because of aberrant drug-related behavior. This trial further demonstrated that substantial improvement in compliance with prescription opioids for many high-risk pain patients is possible within a pain management center.

Screening Results for the Case

Mr. Smith was seen by the treating physician and participated in an initial history and physical examination. He completed a comprehensive pain questionnaire and the SOAPP-R and COMM. He also agreed to give a urine sample for a toxicology screen. He scored a 38 on the SOAPP-R, which was well above the cutoff of 18. He scored a 12 on the COMM, which was again above the cutoff of 9, suggesting risk of medication misuse. His urine toxicology screen showed evidence of morphine and THC, but no signs of oxycodone as he had initially reported.

Ethical Issues

There are a number of ethical considerations worth mentioning in this case. First is the need to prevent harm. Prescription opioids have the potential to contribute to significant harm including intentional or accidental death by overdose and potential problems related to addiction and dependency. Prescription opioid analgesics are among the most frequently abused prescription drugs, and all measures are needed to reduce patient risk including professional training and patient education and counseling.[58,59] More Americans abuse prescription opioids than use cocaine, hallucinogens, inhalants, and heroin combined, and most physicians prescribing pain medication have had no training in addiction issues. For these reasons, clinical and ethical concerns persist about prescribing opioids for chronic noncancer pain.

Second, however, it has been estimated that over 100 million US adults live with moderate to severe pain at any one time and pain is frequently undertreated.[60,61] Forty to 50% of patients with metastatic disease and 90% of patients with terminal cancer have reported severe pain.[60] Thus, there is a very real need to help manage pain and suffering. It is also known that certain patients are denied treatment because of their past history. Substance abuse is more prominent in the chronic pain population than in the general population, and chronic pain patients with psychiatric and substance abuse history have a greater potential for inadequate treatment of pain. Further concerns arise when the patients present with significant comorbid medical concerns.[62] These patients tend to be the most challenging, and there is a need for ongoing discussion of ethical principles regarding the best and most humane ways to help manage pain and suffering while avoiding placing patients in further harm. Carefully following treatment guidelines for responsible opioid prescribing can help in dealing with these troubling issues.[58]

Initial Recommendations

All patients should be assessed for level of risk when opioid therapy is being considered. Ideally, the results of a validated self-report screening tool, urine screen, past history from a previous provider, and history of substance abuse and psychiatric comorbidity are needed to establish level of risk. Patients can be classified according to their risk, and the course of treatment would be determined based on this level.

High-Risk Patients

As can be seen from the history and screening results for Mr. Smith, he falls into the category of high risk for substance use disorder related to opioid pain therapy. After very careful consideration and exhaustion of other treatment options, the decision was made to pursue chronic opioid therapy. The patient read and signed an opioid therapy agreement that outlined his responsibilities and the clinic's policies. Past medical records were obtained and, importantly, contact was maintained with previous and current providers. Mr. Smith was advised of the risks for addiction and was told that he was initially expected to give a urine sample for a toxicology screen to be repeated every clinic visit. He was given medication for limited periods of time (e.g., every 1 to 2 weeks). In this case, his family members were also interviewed and were encouraged to be involved in his care. Often for high-risk subjects, input and counseling from an addiction medicine specialist and/or mental health professional should be sought.

Moderate-Risk Patients

Patients in the moderate-risk category have the potential for substance misuse and subsequent abuse. They should read and sign an opioid therapy agreement. Periodic urine screens should be performed preferably using a surprise, or "random," schedule. After a period in which no signs of aberrant behavior are observed, less frequent clinic visits than monthly, progressing up to every 3 months, may be adequate. If there are any violations of the opioid agreement, then more frequent urine screens and shorter-interval clinic visits are recommended. After two or more violations of the opioid agreement, an assessment by an addiction medicine specialist and/or mental health professional should be mandated. After repeat violations, referral to a substance abuse program could be recommended. A recurrent history of violations would also be grounds for tapering and discontinuing opioid therapy.

Low-Risk Patients

These patients are least likely to develop a substance abuse disorder. Patients should sign an opioid therapy agreement, and after an initial toxicology screen, frequent urine screens would not be indicated. Less worry is needed about the type of opioid to be prescribed and the frequency of clinic visits. Efficacy of opioid therapy should be reassessed every 6 months; urine toxicology screens and an updated opioid therapy agreement would be recommended annually.

Long-Term Plan

Early signs of aberrant behavior and a violation of the opioid agreement can be grounds to taper the medication and possibly refer to a substance abuse program. If the behaviors persist, these patients would be informed that they would not be candidates for opioid therapy but could still receive nonopioid pain therapy. This would need to be well documented. Patients showing minimal efficacy of opioid therapy may also be tapered off their medication. Finally, those high-risk patients who show benefit of treatment and minimal signs of aberrant drug-related behavior over the course of 12 months may require less vigilant monitoring, but tracking progress would always be needed.

Mr. Smith was perceived to be very high risk for medication misuse despite his insistence that he would be responsible with his opioids. After completing a comprehensive review and meeting with providers in an interdisciplinary setting, he was prescribed sustained-release morphine and signed an opioid agreement. His wife agreed to help in monitoring his medication. He was instructed that he would be given doses lasting for 1 week at a time for the first month and that he would need to complete a compliance checklist and give a urine sample during each clinic visit. He was told that he would have to refrain from using marijuana. He was also requested to meet with a psychologist once a month for motivational counseling regarding his pain and substance use.

Over the course of a year, Mr. Smith was compliant in the use of this medication. He did not show signs of any aberrant drug-related behavior. He was maintained on a steady dose of opioids while also taking advantage of adjuvant medications and treatments. He also met with a physical therapist with specialty training in pain management. He eventually was retrained as a codes inspector and continued to work part time through his local city council while being maintained on stable doses of opioids.

Summary Points

Comprehensive assessment and monitoring are recommended for all patients who are being considered for long-term opioid therapy for chronic pain. The close monitoring of patients who are at greatest risk for misuse of their prescribed medication should contain a treatment protocol that includes an opioid agreement, regular urine toxicology screens, compliance checklists, pill counts, and, if indicated, motivational counseling. Careful monitoring and use of abuse-deterrent opioids will hopefully decrease the abuse potential of prescribed opioids. Risk of opioid misuse and addiction will remain, and close attention to screening and documentation of treatment outcomes will continue to be the gold standard of opioid therapy.

Acknowledgments

This work was supported in part by a grant from the National Institute on Drug Abuse (NIDA) of the National Institutes of Health, Bethesda, MD (R21 DA024298, Jamison, PI).

References

1. Andersson GBJ. Epidemiological features of low back pain. *Lancet.* 1999;354:581–585.

2. Bair M, Robinson R, Katon W, Kroenke K. Depression and pain comorbidity: a literature review. *Arch Int Med.* 2003;163:2433–2445.

3. Peloso PM, Bellamy N, Bensen W, et al. Double blind randomized placebo control trial of controlled release codeine in the treatment of osteoarthritis of the hip or knee. *J Rheumatol Suppl.* 2000;27(3):764–771.

4. Katz JN, Stucki G, Lipson SJ, Fossel AH, Grobler LJ, Weinstein JN. Predictors of surgical outcome in degenerative lumbar spinal stenosis. *Spine.* 1999;24(21):2229–2233.

5. Katz JN, Lipson SJ, Lew RA, et al. Lumbar laminectomy alone or with instrumented or noninstrumented arthrodesis in degenerative lumbar spinal stenosis: patient selection, costs, and surgical outcomes. *Spine.* 1997;22(10):1123–1131.

6. Caldwell J, Hale M, Boyd R, et al. Treatment of osteoarthritis pain with controlled release oxycodone or fixed combination oxycodone plus acetaminophen added to nonsteroidal antiinflammatory drugs: a double blind, randomized, multicenter, placebo controlled trial. *J Rheum.* 1999;26(4):862–869.

7. Maier C, Hildebrandt J, Klinger R, Henrich-Eberl C, Lindena G. Morphine responsiveness, efficacy and tolerability in patients with chronic non-tumor pain—results of a double-blind placebo-controlled trial (MONTAS). *Pain.* 2002;97(3):223–233.

8. Kalso E, Edwards JE, Moore RA, McQuay HJ. Opioids in chronic non-cancer pain: systematic review of efficacy and safety. *Pain.* 2004;112(3):372–380.

9. von Korff M, Deyo RA. Potent opioids for chronic musculoskeletal pain: flying blind? *Pain.* 2004;109(3):207–209.

10. Arkinstall W, Sandler A, Goughnour B, Babul N, Harsanyl Z, Darke AC. Efficacy of controlled-release codeine in chronic non-malignant pain: a randomized, placebo-controlled clinical trial. *Pain.* 1995;62(2):169–178.

11. Breckenridge J, Clark J. Patient characteristics associated with opioid vs. nonsteroidal anti-inflammatory drug management of chronic low back pain. *J Pain.* 2003;4(6):344–350.

12. Moulin DE, Iezzi A, Amireh R, Sharpe WKJ, Boyd D, Merskey H. Randomized trial of oral morphine for chronic non-cancer pain. *Lancet.* 1996;347:143–147.

13. Rivest C, Katz JN, Ferrante FM, Jamison RN. Effects of epidural steroid injection on pain due to lumbar spinal stenosis or herniated disks: a prospective study. *Arthritis Care Res.* 1998;11(4):291–297.

14. Rooks DS, Huang J, Bierbaum BE, et al. The effect of preoperative exercise on measures of functional status in men and women undergoing total hip and knee arthroplasty. *Arthritis Care Res.* 2006;55(5):700–708.

15. Rakvag TT, Klepstad P, Baar C, et al. The Val 158Met polymorphism of the human catechol-O-methyltransferase (COMT) gene may influence morphine requirements in cancer pain patients. *Pain.* 2005;116:73–78.

16. Wasan AD, Kaptchuk TJ, Davar G, Jamison RN. The association between psychopathology and placebo analgesia in patients with discogenic low back pain. *Pain Med.* 2006;7(3):217–228.

17. Boersma K, Linton SJ. Screening to identify patients at risk: profiles of psychological risk factors for early intervention. *Clin J Pain.* 2005;21(1):38–43.

18. Fishbain D. Approaches to treatment decisions for psychiatric comorbidity in the management of the chronic pain patient. *Med Clin North Am.* 1999;83(3):737–759.

19. Wasan AD, Davar G, Jamison RN. The association between negative affect and opioid analgesia in patients with discogenic low back pain. *Pain.* 2005;117:450–461.

20. Kessler R, McGonagle K, Zhao S. Lifetime and 12-month prevalence of DSM-III-R psychiatric disorders in the Unites States: results from the National Comorbidity Survey. *Arch Gen Psychiatry.* 1994;51:8–19.

21. Cornelius J, Salloum I, Ehler J. Fluoxetine in depressed alcoholics: a double-blind, placebo-controlled trial. *Arch Gen Psychiatry.* 1997;54:700–705.

22. Sonne S, Brady K. Substance abuse and bipolar comorbidity. *Psychiatry Clin North Am.* 1999;22:609–627.

23. Brady KT, Myrick H, Sonne S. Comorbid addiction and affective disorders. In: Graham AW, Schultz TK, Wilford BB, eds. Principles of Addiction Medicine. 2nd ed. Arlington, VA: American Society of Addiction Medicine; 1998. pp. 983–992.

24. Hasin D, Liu X, Nunes E. Effects of major depression on remission and relapse of substance dependence. *Arch Gen Psychiatry.* 2002;59:375–380.

25. Quello S, Brady K, Sonne S. Mood disorders and substance use disorder: a complex comorbidity. *NIDA Science Pract Prespect.* 2005;3:13–24.

26. Gilson AM, Ryan KM, Joranson DE, Dahl JL. A reassessment of trends in the medical use and abuse of opioid analgesics and implications for diversion control: 1997–2002. *J Pain Symptom Manage.* 2004;28(2):176–188.

27. American Academy of Pain Medicine, the American Pain Society, the American Society of Addiction Medicine. *Definitions related to the use of opioids for the treatment of pain: a consensus document from the American Academy of Pain Medicine, the American Pain Society, and the American Society of Addiction Medicine.* Chevy Chase, MD: ASAM; 2001.

28. *American Psychiatric Association. Diagnostic and statistical manual of mental disorders.* 4th ed. Washington, DC: American Psychiatric Association; 1994.

29. Leshner A. What does it mean that addiction is a brain disease? *Monitor Psychol.* 2001;32:19.

30. Department of Justice. Dispensing controlled substances for the treatment of pain. Federal Register Notices 2006. DEA-286P. Available from: http://www.deadiversion.usdoj.gov/fed_regs/notices/2006/fr09062.htm. Accessed September 24, 2012.

31. Hampton T. Experts point to lessons learned from controversy over rofecoxib safety. *JAMA.* 2005;293:413–414.

32. McNairy SL, Maruta T, Ivnik RJ, Swanson DW, Ilstrup DW. Prescription medication dependence and neuropsychologic function. *Pain.* 1984;18:169–177.

33. Darton LA, Dilts SL. Opioids. In: Frances RJ, Miller SL, eds. *Clinical textbook of addictive disorders.* 2nd ed. New York: Guilford Press; 1998.

34. Savage SR. Addiction in the treatment of pain: significance, recognition, and management. *J Pain Symptom Manage.* 1993;8:265–278.

35. Jamison RN, Link CL, Marceau LD. Do pain patients at high risk for substance misuse experience more pain?: a longitudinal outcomes study. *Pain Med.* 2009;10(6):1084–1094.

36. Jamison RN, Butler SF, Budman SH, Edwards RR, Wasan AD. Gender differences in risk factors for aberrant prescription opioid use. *J Pain.* 2010;11(4):312–320.

37. Robinson RC, Gatchel RJ, Polatin P, Deschner M, Noe C, Gajraj N. Screening for problematic prescription opioid use. *Clin J Pain.* 2001;17:220–228.

38. Helzer JE, Robins LN. The Diagnostic Interview Schedule: its development, evaluations, and use. *Soc Psychiatry Psychiatric Epidem.* 1988;23:6–16.

39. Mayfield D, Mcleod G, Hall P. The CAGE questionnaire: validation of a new alcoholism screening instrument. *Am J Psychiatry.* 1974;131:1121–1123.

40. Selzer M. The Michigan alcoholism screening test: the quest for a new diagnostic instrument. *Am J Psychiatry.* 1971;127:1653–1658.

41. Webster LR, Webster RM. Predicting aberrant behaviors in opioid-treated patients: preliminary validation of the Opioid Risk Tool. *Pain Med.* 2005;6(6):432–442.

42. Butler SF, Budman SH, Fernandez K, Jamison RN. Validation of a screener and opioid assessment measure for patients with chronic pain. *Pain.* 2004;112(1–2):65–75.

43. Butler SF, Fernandez K, Benoit C, Budman SH, Jamison RN. Validation of the revised Screener and Opioid Assessment for Patients with Pain (SOAPP-R). *J Pain.* 2008;9(4):360–372.

44. Butler SF, Budman SH, Fernandez K C, Fanciullo GJ, Jamison RN. Cross-validation of a screener to predict opioid misuse in chronic pain patients. *J Addict Med.* 2009;3:66–73.

45. Butler SF, Budman SH, Fernandez KC, et al. Development and validation of the Current Opioid Misuse Measure. *Pain.* 2007;130(1–2):144–156.

46. Butler SF, Budman SH, Fanciullo GJ, Jamison R. Cross Validation of the Current Opioid Misuse Measure (COMM) to monitor chronic pain patients on opioid therapy. *Clin J Pain.* 2010;26:770–776.

47. Webster LR, Dove B. *Avoiding Opioid Abuse While Managing Pain: A Guide for Practitioners.* North Branch, MN: Sunrise River Press; 2007.

48. Belgrade M. The DIRE Score: predicting outcomes of opioid prescribing for chronic pain. *J Pain.* 2006;7:671–681.

49. Passik SD, Kirsch KL, Whitcomb RK, et al. A new tool to assess and document pain outcomes in chronic pain patients receiving opioid therapy. *Clin Ther.* 2004;26(4):552–561.

50. Coambs RB, Jarry JL, Santhiapillai AS, Abrahamsohn RV, Atance CM. The SISAP: a new screening instrument for identifying potential opioid abusers in the management of chronic malignant pain within general medical practice. *Pain Res Manage.* 1996;1:155–162.

51. Fishbain DA, Cutler RB, Rosomoff HL, Rosomoff RS. Validity of self-reported drug use in chronic pain patients. *Clin J Pain.* 1999;15(3):184–191.

52. Michna E, Jamison RN, Pham LD, et al. Urine toxicology screening among chronic pain patients on opioid therapy: frequency and predictability of abnormal findings. *Clin J Pain.* 2007;23(2):173–179.

53. Katz NP, Fanciullo GJ. Role of urine toxicology testing in the management of chronic opioid therapy. *Clin J Pain.* 2002;18(4 Suppl):S76–S82.

54. Reisfield GM, Salazar E, Bertholf RL. Rational use and interpretation of urine drug testing in chronic opioid therapy. *Ann Clin Lab Sci.* 2007;37:301–314.

55. Reisfield GM, Wasan AD, Jamison RN. The prevalence and significance of cannabis use in patients prescribed chronic opioid therapy: a review of the extant literature. *Pain Med.* 2009;10:1434–1441.

56. Munsey C. Medicine or menace: psychologists' research can inform the growing debate over legalizing marijuana. *Monitor Psychol.* 2010;41(6):50–55.

57. Jamison RN, Ross EL, Michna E, Chen LQ, Holcomb C, Wasan AD. Substance misuse treatment for high-risk chronic pain patients on opioid therapy: a randomized trial. *Pain.* 2010;150:390–400.

58. Chou R, Fanciullo GJ, Fine P, et al. Clinical guidelines for the use of chronic opioid therapy in noncancer pain. *J Pain.* 2009;10:113–130.

59. Food and Drug Administration. Opioid drugs and risk evaluation and mitigation strategies. 2011. http://www.fda.gov/drugs/drugsafety/informationbydrugclass/ucm163647.htm. Accessed on September 24, 2012.

60. Rosenblum A, Joseph H, Fong C, Kipnis S, Cleeland C, Portenoy R. Prevalence and characteristics of chronic pain among chemically dependent patients in methadone maintenance and residential treatment facilities. *JAMA.* 2003;289:2370–2378.

61. Institute of Medicine. *Relieving pain in America: A blueprint for transforming prevention, care, education, and research.* Consensus report released June 29, 2011. http://ion.edu/Reports/2011.

62. Chiauzzi E, Traudeau KJ, Zacharoff K, Bond K. Identifying primary care skills and competencies in opioid risk management. *J Cont Ed Health Prof.* 2011;31:231–240.

Chapter 4

Functional Pain Syndromes

Claudia Sommer, Nurcan Üçeyler

The Case

Susanne Adam, a 57-year-old woman, first noticed fatigue and reduced working performance at the age of 42 with diminished alertness and difficulties in concentration. She also developed pain in the extremities that was initially changing in location and intensity. Until then she had never been seriously ill. However, within 2 years the muscle pain became permanent in the arms and then also in the legs. Symptoms rapidly progressed with additional complaints such as alternating episodes of diarrhea and obstipation, and urge incontinence. These gastrointestinal and bladder symptoms were followed by the occurrence of daily headache and severe sleep disturbances with less than 4 hours of nonrefreshing sleep per night. From the age of 49 years, Ms. Adam was no longer able to work full time as a geriatric nurse, and 1 year later fibromyalgia syndrome (FMS) was diagnosed. She then took part in a mind–body rehabilitation program that she considered beneficial. However, she was still unable to return to work.

Ms. Adam's current complaints were permanent and deep muscle pain and the feeling of muscle stiffness. Pain was located in all muscles but mainly in the upper arms and thighs. The pain character was described as aching and pressing and mean pain intensity was estimated as 5/10 with a maximum of 8/10. Pressure to the muscles and physical activities such as carrying bags exacerbated her pain, and exercises such as walking and gymnastics relieved her pain. Ms. Adam reported that she was able to handle her housework without help; however, she needed frequent breaks. Sleep disturbance was still a major complaint, as were bladder and gastrointestinal symptoms, the latter especially during emotional stress. Although Ms. Adam reported stable mood with only rare and mild episodes of depressive symptoms, she received psychological treatment regularly, which improved coping. She also had developed effective coping strategies such as distracting herself with hobbies.

Pharmacologic treatment had been started with a cyclooxygenase-2 (COX2) inhibitor (etoricoxib), which provided mild pain relief. This treatment was stopped when the patient became fearful of potential side effects of

COX2 inhibitors. Other nonsteroidal anti-inflammatory drugs (NSAIDs) such as diclofenac were ineffective. The patient was then put on weak opioids, starting with tramadol 100 mg/day. However, a few days later side effects including dizziness, vertigo, and increased fatigue occurred while pain was not reduced. Another trial with retarded tilidine/naloxone 50/4 mg/day had the same outcome and medication had to be stopped after a few weeks. Slow-release oxycodone, a strong opioid, was started at a dose of 20 mg bid and increased to 40 mg bid over 4 weeks. A laxative and an antiemetic were given to counteract side effects. However, no effect on pain severity was observed and the medication was again stopped. The patient was then put on trimipramine 25 mg/day, which slightly relieved pain without too many side effects.

List of Considerations

- Opioid suitability for fibromyalgia, other functional pain syndromes, and other conditions with no organic cause
- Risk versus benefit of opioids in this case
- Responding to a failed opioid trial

Clinical Discussion

This patient with FMS had an initial response to a COX2 inhibitor but not to a nonselective COX inhibitor. In accordance with the World Health Organization (WHO) ladder, a weak opioid was then given, and later a strong opioid. None of these drugs was convincingly effective. The WHO ladder was developed for cancer pain, and modifications for noncancer pain have been suggested.[1] However, many years of experience with the WHO ladder have brought about its use also in noncancer pain.

Although up to 50% of patients with FMS are treated with opioids,[2,3] there is evidence only for tramadol (a weak opioid μ agonist with modest serotonin nonspecific reuptake inhibition) use in FMS.[4,5] Because the present patient's complaints started with a musculoskeletal type of pain with varying localization, indicative of strain-related pain due to her job as a geriatric nurse, it is reasonable that her initial treatment consisted of a COX2 inhibitor and nonselective NSAIDs. In fact, up to 40% of FMS patients take NSAIDs or have taken them in the course of their disease.[6,7] Four randomized controlled trials (RCTs) have been published including 181 FMS patients with a mean treatment duration of 5 weeks. The trials were of low methodologic quality. Three of them were performed with ibuprofen, one with tenoxicam. COX2 inhibitors have not been tested in RCTs in FMS yet. Ibuprofen and tenoxicam were no better than placebo in these trials. Although NSAIDs are commonly used, especially early in the course of FMS, some national guidelines do not recommend the use of either standard NSAIDs or selective COX2 inhibitors in FMS.[8] Others do favor the use of NSAIDs in FMS. The European League Against Rheumatism (EULAR) recommends simple analgesics such as acetaminophen on the basis of expert opinion.[9] NSAIDs may have a synergistic effect when combined with centrally active agents such as tricyclic antidepressants and anticonvulsants.[10] In a survey of 1,042 FMS patients, 66.1% stated that they found NSAIDs more effective than acetaminophen.[11] Because simple analgesics and NSAIDs have an acceptable side effect profile, some experts recommend including them in the management of FMS despite the lack of conclusive evidence and the risk of significant cardiovascular, renal, and gastrointestinal side effects.[12]

Tramadol is the only opioid that has been tested for FMS pain in an RCT. Tramadol is not only a weak μ agonist but also a noradrenalin and serotonin reuptake inhibitor. Tramadol in combination with acetaminophen was tested in a group of 384 patients; the mean duration of treatment was 9.5 weeks.[4,5] The quality of the study was medium; the effect sizes on pain and quality of life at the end of the study were small. Patient acceptance was low, with a dropout rate of 40%, which was, however, lower than that of placebo.

None of the strong opioids has been tested in RCTs in FMS. In an open case series, a fentanyl patch (25 μg/72 hours) was given to 12 FMS patients over 4 to 8 weeks. None of the patients had a significant reduction in pain or an increase in quality of life. All patients had side effects such as confusion, nausea, and vomiting. Seven of 16 dropped out of the study prematurely.[13] In a small RCT with nine FMS patients who received 10 mg of intravenous morphine hydrochloride, there was no effect compared to placebo. However, side effects such as nausea and vomiting were prominent. In a nonrandomized trial of 4 years' duration with 38 FMS patients receiving opioids, which was only published in abstract form, there was no significant alleviation of pain over time.[14]

It has been hypothesized that the lack of efficacy of opioids in FMS is related to alterations in endogenous opioid activity. In a positron emission tomography (PET) study using a selective ligand for the μ-opioid receptor (MOR), MOR binding potential in several brain regions implicated in pain modulation, including the nucleus accumbens, the amygdala, and the dorsal cingulate, was reduced.[15] Reduced MOR binding potential has since been observed in complex regional pain syndrome, another chronic pain condition with little effect of opioids.[16] This finding may be interpreted as a sign of endogenous opioid analgesic activity, which would then reduce the efficacy of exogenous opioids in one of two ways: Either there is decreased MOR binding potential because the receptors are occupied by endogenous opioids, or the MOR may be down-regulated after prolonged stimulation. However, findings of a recent experiment with the opioid antagonist naltrexone did not confirm an altered function of the endogenous opioid system in women with FMS.[17] Intriguingly, another group found an up-regulation of δ-opioid receptors (DORs) and κ-opioid receptors (KORs) in the skin of FMS patients[18]; the significance of this finding is still unclear.

If opioid drugs are not effective in patients with FMS but have been given for a long period of time, drug withdrawal may be needed. In a group of 159

FMS patients admitted to a rehabilitation program, 38% took opioids at admission, and only 3% at discharge 3 weeks later. Pain and quality-of-life scores were better after withdrawal than before.[19]

Some authors group FMS together with temporomandibular dysfunction (TMD), vulvodynia, irritable bowel syndrome (IBS), and chronic pelvic pain (painful bladder, interstitial cystitis) as functional pain disorders or central sensitivity disorders.[20–22] There are no RCTs of opioid use in these conditions. Expert opinion has supported the use of opioids in a subset of TMD patients.[23] Opioids may be used in IBS, if diarrhea is a dominant symptom, but are not otherwise commonly used in this condition, especially where severe obstipation is already a problem. There is an interesting observation that there is an increased MOR expression in ileal and colonic enteric neurons in IBS, and that a selective peripheral MOR agonist could modulate the production of tumor necrosis factor-α (TNF-α) in colonic organ cultures.[24] Whether this translates to the clinic is as yet unknown. For chronic pelvic pain, again there are no RCTs, and experts support the use of opioids "for pain control under adequate supervision."[25]

Patients with FMS do not necessarily seek opioid treatment for their pain. Given the evidence that opioid efficacy is limited and side effects often poorly tolerated in these patients, it is reasonable to consider opioids a treatment of last resort for FMS. Many FMS patients prefer nonmedical treatment options and mostly report on the long-term efficacy of physical activity. Although exercise may initially increase the muscular symptoms, many patients report pain relief afterward. In fact, exercise-based programs of mild to moderate intensity with a frequency of 2 or 3 times per week are efficacious in reducing pain and depression and in improving physical fitness in FMS patients.[26,27] Furthermore, psychological therapy, in particular cognitive behavioral treatment, has small but robust effects.[28]

Ethical Issues

With little evidence that strong opioids may be beneficial in patients with FMS, it is best to avoid their prescription. On the other hand, in a patient suffering from severe pain, and when other options have not been successful, it may as well be unethical to withhold opioid treatment.[29] It has been proposed to employ patient-centered principles, which include negotiating treatment goals, avoiding harm, and incorporating chronic opioids into the treatment plan only if they improve the patient's overall health-related quality of life.[30] In any case, this can only be done after clearly explaining the potential risks and benefits to the patient; most important, the will of the patient needs to be respected, and in many cases FMS patients initially treated with opioids prefer to discontinue their use. Furthermore, if the opioid is not effective, it should be withdrawn before long-term use makes withdrawal more difficult. Rather than being prescribed an opioid, FMS patients should be informed about the treatment options that are more likely successful long term.

Initial Recommendations

Once Ms. Adam's FMS was diagnosed, the primary aims of her therapy were improvement of function and alleviation of and adaptation to the symptoms. Choice of treatment options should respect her preferences after information about the syndrome and the possibilities and limitations of the different treatment options were presented to her. Patient education and aerobic exercise should be early nonpharmacologic steps.

Long-Term Plan

Cognitive behavioral therapy may help to develop or improve Ms. Adam's coping strategies. Because her pain failed to improve on opioids, other drugs that have shown efficacy in FMS may be prescribed, although the effect sizes are usually small. These drugs mainly belong to the classes of antidepressants[31] and calcium channel anticonvulsants.[32] Among these, duloxetine, pregabalin, and milnacipran have been approved by the US Food and Drug Administration (FDA) for FMS.[33] Depending on comorbidities and contraindications, the patient might be given one of these drugs.

Summary Points

- Opioids should be avoided in functional pain syndromes like FMS
- Opioids may be used on a trial basis for pain exacerbations, but should be withdrawn if not efficacious or if the exacerbation has remitted.
- A combination of patient education, physical therapy, physiotherapy, cognitive behavioral therapy, and evidence based non-opioid pharmacotherapy may be more adequate.

References

1. Vargas-Schaffer G. Is the WHO analgesic ladder still valid? Twenty-four years of experience. *Can Fam Physician.* 2010;56:514–517, e202–e205.

2. Berger A, Sadosky A, Dukes EM, Edelsberg J, Zlateva G, Oster G. Patterns of healthcare utilization and cost in patients with newly diagnosed fibromyalgia. *Am J Manag Care.* 2010;16:S126–S137.

3. White LA, Robinson RL, Yu AP, et al. Comparison of health care use and costs in newly diagnosed and established patients with fibromyalgia. *J Pain.* 2009;10:976–983.

4. Bennett RM, Kamin M, Karim R, Rosenthal N. Tramadol and acetaminophen combination tablets in the treatment of fibromyalgia pain: a double-blind, randomized, placebo-controlled study. *Am J Med.* 2003;114:537–545.

5. Russell IJ, Kamin M, Bennett RM, Schnitzer TJ, Green JA, Katz WA. Efficacy of tramadol in treatment of pain in fibromyalgia. *J Clin Rheumatol.* 2000;6:250–257.

6. Bennett RM, Jones J, Turk DC, Russell IJ, Matallana L. An internet survey of 2,596 people with fibromyalgia. *BMC Musculoskelet Disord.* 2007;8:27.

7. Müller A, Hartmann M, Eich W. [Health care utilization in patients with Fibromyalgia Syndrome (FMS)]. *Schmerz.* 2000;14:77–83.

8. Häuser W, Klose P, Langhorst J, et al. Efficacy of different types of aerobic exercise in fibromyalgia syndrome: a systematic review and meta-analysis of randomised controlled trials. *Arthritis Res Ther.* 2010;12:R79.

9. Carville SF, Arendt-Nielsen S, Bliddal H, et al. EULAR evidence-based recommendations for the management of fibromyalgia syndrome. *Ann Rheum Dis.* 2008;67:536–541.

10. Goldenberg DL, Felson DT, Dinerman H. A randomized, controlled trial of amitriptyline and naproxen in the treatment of patients with fibromyalgia. *Arthritis Rheum.* 1986;29:1371–1377.

11. Wolfe F, Zhao S, Lane N. Preference for nonsteroidal antiinflammatory drugs over acetaminophen by rheumatic disease patients: a survey of 1,799 patients with osteoarthritis, rheumatoid arthritis, and fibromyalgia. *Arthritis Rheum.* 2000;43:378–385.

12. Ngian GS, Guymer EK, Littlejohn GO. The use of opioids in fibromyalgia. *Int J Rheum Dis.* 2011;14:6–11.

13. Callejas Rubio JL, Fernandez Moyano A, Navarro Hidalgo D, Palmero Palmero C. [Percutaneous fentanyl in fibromyalgia]. *Med Clin (Barc).* 2003;120:358–359.

14. Kemple KL, Smith G, Wong-Ngan J. Opioid therapy in fibromyalgia: a four year prospective evaluation of therapy selection, efficacy, and predictions of outcome. *Arthritis Rheum.* 2003;48:S88.

15. Harris RE, Clauw DJ, Scott DJ, McLean SA, Gracely RH, Zubieta JK. Decreased central mu-opioid receptor availability in fibromyalgia. *J Neurosci.* 2007;27:10000–10006.

16. Klega A, Eberle T, Buchholz HG, et al. Central opioidergic neurotransmission in complex regional pain syndrome. *Neurology.* 2010;75:129–136.

17. Younger JW, Zautra AJ, Cummins ET. Effects of naltrexone on pain sensitivity and mood in fibromyalgia: no evidence for endogenous opioid pathophysiology. *PLoS One.* 2009;4:e5180.

18. Salemi S, Aeschlimann A, Wollina U, et al. Up-regulation of delta-opioid receptors and kappa-opioid receptors in the skin of fibromyalgia patients. *Arthritis Rheum.* 2007;56:2464–2466.

19. Hooten WM, Townsend CO, Sletten CD, Bruce BK, Rome JD. Treatment outcomes after multidisciplinary pain rehabilitation with analgesic medication withdrawal for patients with fibromyalgia. *Pain Med.* 2007;8:8–16.

20. Bradley LA. Pathophysiologic mechanisms of fibromyalgia and its related disorders. *J Clin Psychiatry.* 2008;69(Suppl 2):6–13.

21. Kindler LL, Bennett RM, Jones KD. Central sensitivity syndromes: mounting pathophysiologic evidence to link fibromyalgia with other common chronic pain disorders. *Pain Manag Nurs.* 2011;12:15–24.

22. Persu C, Cauni V, Gutue S, Blaj I, Jinga V, Geavlete P. From interstitial cystitis to chronic pelvic pain. *J Med Life.* 2010;3:167–174.

23. Bouloux GF. Use of opioids in long-term management of temporomandibular joint dysfunction. *J Oral Maxillofac Surg.* 2011;69:1885–1891.

24. Philippe D, Chakass D, Thuru X, et al. Mu opioid receptor expression is increased in inflammatory bowel diseases: implications for homeostatic intestinal inflammation. *Gut.* 2006;55:815–823.

25. Jarrell JF, Vilos GA, Allaire C, et al. Consensus guidelines for the management of chronic pelvic pain. *J Obstet Gynaecol Can.* 2005;27:869–910.

26. Busch AJ, Webber SC, Brachaniec M, et al. Exercise therapy for fibromyalgia. *Curr Pain Headache Rep.* 2011;15:358–367.

27. Häuser W, Petzke F, Sommer C. Comparative efficacy and harms of duloxetine, milnacipran, and pregabalin in fibromyalgia syndrome. *J Pain.* 2010;11:505–521.

28. Glombiewski JA, Sawyer AT, Gutermann J, Koenig K, Rief W, Hofmann SG. Psychological treatments for fibromyalgia: a meta-analysis. *Pain.* 2010;151:280–295.

29. Ballantyne JC, Fleisher LA. Ethical issues in opioid prescribing for chronic pain. *Pain.* 2010;148:365–367.

30. Sullivan M, Ferrell B. Ethical challenges in the management of chronic nonmalignant pain: negotiating through the cloud of doubt. *J Pain.* 2005;6:2–9.

31. Häuser W, Bernardy K, Üçeyler N, Sommer C. Treatment of fibromyalgia syndrome with antidepressants: a meta-analysis. *JAMA.* 2009;301:198–209.

32. Häuser W, Bernardy K, Üçeyler N, Sommer C. Treatment of fibromyalgia syndrome with gabapentin and pregabalin—a meta-analysis of randomized controlled trials. *Pain.* 2009;145:69–81.

33. Häuser W, Thieme K, Turk DC. Guidelines on the management of fibromyalgia syndrome—a systematic review. *Eur J Pain.* 2010;14:5–10.

Chapter 5

Chronic Opioid Therapy in Childhood and Adolescence

Lisa Isaac, Stephen C. Brown, Jennifer Tyrrell,
Patricia A. McGrath

The Case

Cassie is a 13-year-old girl with back pain after scoliosis surgery. She is now 1 year post–posterior scoliosis repair. Pain is constant, aching, throbbing, and in multiple sites including the neck and upper and lower back. Usual pain is rated as 7/10, with a range of 5 to 10/10, and pain is the worst in the mornings and late evenings.

Pain produces significant disruption to sports—she was previously in a high-level gymnastics training school—requiring a change in schools, which had a marked impact on her academic performance. She has diminished time with friends (by about 40%), and she sleeps poorly. She can't find a comfortable position in which to fall asleep and she awakens 2 to 3 times per night.

She is the youngest of three children, living with both parents. Her mother has chronic back pain, is on long-term disability, and uses a fentanyl patch for pain management.

Blood work, electromyelography (EMG), and x-ray results were normal. No source of infection could be found.

Treatments tried include nonsteroidal anti-inflammatory drugs (NSAIDs), which resulted in gastrointestinal (GI) upset and bleed; acetaminophen was ineffective; gabapentin, pregabalin, amitriptyline, and carbamazepine were all ineffective despite adequate trials; and tramadol caused nausea. Cassie was unable to comply with graded exercise because of pain. Family finances and distance from the hospital have made consistent psychosocial support minimal, but relaxation tapes have been unhelpful.

List of Considerations

- Adolescents (and children) may have difficulty distinguishing emotional effects of opioids; they may be vulnerable to difficulty determining the best balance of adverse effects versus benefits

- Poor concentration (driving is poorly established in this age group, so the concern of decreased reflexes becomes more relevant)
- Alteration of the hypothalamic-pituitary axis (especially hypogonadism, but possibly decreased sexual drive, increased thyroid-stimulating hormone, and altered luteinizing hormone secretion resulting in altered development of puberty)[1]
- Parental concerns regarding opioid use (misconceptions, etc.)
- Storage of the medications and administration at school
- Peer and sibling pressure/misconceptions
- Nature and frequency of monitoring; the child is dependent on others to travel to appointments
- Sleep architecture may be altered[2]
- Tolerance and increased dosing (adolescents may be at increased risk of tolerance to opioids)[3]
- Motivation and gratification neurologic circuitry change during adolescence and may be altered with opioid administration;[5,6] may increase risk for substance abuse[7]
- Potential risk for addiction, particularly for adolescents[8] (20% of adolescents will try prescription drugs for nonmedical use[9])
- Ability to assess compliance and potential drug abuse[4,10]
- Unknown long-term consequences on physical, cognitive, and social health and development; long-term effects of opioids are not clearly understood in this population.

Clinical Discussion

Treatment decisions regarding the use of opioid medication for the management of nonmalignant chronic pain in children are complicated by many of the considerations presented throughout this text, as well as by developmental, family, societal, and ethical considerations unique to children and adolescents. In this chapter, we use a case history of a preteen with complex chronic pain to describe the critical deliberations involved in using opioids with children.

The use of opioids for the management of chronic noncancer pain in children remains controversial due to concerns about dependence and addiction, effects on the undeveloped brain, and effects on development, including intellectual development and education, among other concerns (for review see [11]). While there is now more consensus on the use of opioids for certain chronic pain conditions such as painful sickle cell crises, epidermolysis bullosa, and osteogenesis imperfecta, many questions remain about using opioids chronically in children and adolescents. Yet, the lack of data about the long-term impact of opioid use for noncancer pain in children has prevented us from developing child-centered guidelines for use in clinical practice. Instead, our treatment decisions about when to use opioids to control pain for a child such as Cassie are made on a case-by-case basis gained from our own experience as pediatric pain specialists and the emerging guidelines for opioid use in adults with chronic noncancer pain.

A general outline for opioid decision making is presented in Figure 5.1.

Risk Factors for Opioid Misuse in Adolescents

Adolescents are risk takers, as they are at the developmental stage of determining their own limits and their self-control. Adolescents are more frequently

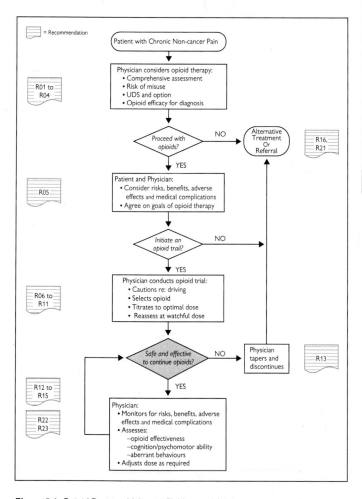

Figure 5.1 Opioid Decision-Making in Children and Adolescents.

risk takers, compared to other age groups, which may increase the risk of substance misuse.[8] They are developing a sense of self and have less reward sensitivity and cognitive control, and thus may have inherently less protection from misusing substances.[12] In addition, 41.7% of students grade 7 and above have tried illicit drugs for nonmedical use in the past year.[13] Whether this increases the risk of future abuse is unclear, although it appears to be unlikely. Twenty percent of adolescents will try prescription opioid drugs for nonmedical use.[9] Alcohol misuse is associated with a higher incidence of other drug misuse, and alcohol misuse may not yet be detected in the teenager. These factors, then, taken together, may increase the chance of using prescription opioids for nonmedical reasons, although not necessarily increase the chance of abuse.

To protect this vulnerable population, the prescriber should feel comfortable with the youth's compliance, use of the medication, and coadministration of other medications. Nevertheless, determining compliance and use of nonprescription drugs may be difficult. In Canada, there are no central databases for tracking of opioids by prescription and patient, such that multiple prescribers are possible. And there is no way of independently verifying nonprescription drug use, other than screening.

Long-Term Consequences of Opioid Use in Adolescents

There are multiple long-term consequences that may be more pertinent for the child or adolescent than the adult. First, cognitive changes or modifications may be relevant for this population, and maybe more than in the adult. Cognitive changes from opioid use in the neonate appear unlikely[14] but possible[15] at age 5, but these studies are limited by testing fatigue in this age group and would benefit from longer-term follow-up. Increasing evidence suggests structural changes in the brain with long-term use of opioids,[5,6] and this may be more significant in the child or adolescent. Endocrine changes particularly relevant to the adolescent include depression of the hypothalamic-pituitary axis. Many rat and some human studies confirm the influence of long-term opioids on hypogonadism and possibly on sexual drive.[1] Finally, the alteration of sleep architecture could have unintended consequences in adolescents, for whom sleep is a vital part of their well-being and physical development.[2] Nevertheless, despite evolving evidence of the long-term effects of opioids on this population, it is important to remember that serious persistent pain can also have a deleterious effect on physical, emotional, intellectual, and social development.

Embarking on Opioids for Life

Population studies in adults strongly suggest that adults treated with opioids continuously (daily) for more than 90 days tend to stay on opioids for prolonged periods, often for life. This is especially true for adults with childhood and other trauma.[16–19] Neuroadaptations such as tolerance and dependence appear to be key factors when it becomes difficult to taper opioids in the face of poor effectiveness.[20] Because neuroadaptations (especially tolerance and dependence) are not easily reversed in children, the high possibility that prolonged opioid therapy (>90 days) could become lifelong should be discussed with children and their parents. This is also a reason to avoid prolonged opioid therapy in young people for all but refractory pain that interferes with function and quality of life.

Monitoring

Monitoring in the child and adolescent is always challenging in that they are dependent on others for help with compliance, including follow-up appointments. Thus, the caregivers are an important part of the management plan and should be included in much of the discussion. They must be implicated in the safekeeping of opioids in the home, particularly when there are younger siblings, as well as in follow-up plans. While the majority of the younger pediatric patients have a low potential for narcotic abuse, this potential exists for adolescent and young adult patients who dispense these medications to themselves. In those patients in whom this may be a concern, a urine drug screening (UDS) test may be employed. We did not feel a UDS was required for Cassie, due to excellent patient compliance, parental oversight, and single prescriber of low-dose opioid. During titration of the opioid to desired effect, untoward side effects are discussed and anticipated. Young adults who are 16 years old or older are instructed not to drive a car until a stable opioid dose has been obtained and potential sedating side effects are not an issue. Cassie is 13 years old, so that was not an issue here. The plan for ongoing monitoring and control of medications and nonprescribed drugs should be open and nonjudgmental. As such, we monitor at least weekly by phone and monthly by visit until an effective dose is established, at which point monitoring can decrease to monthly by phone and visits every 3 months. Prescriptions are dispensed biweekly. Continuity of care and only one prescriber for the patient's opioids are extremely important in the prescribing of opioids in general, but particularly for children and adolescents.

Other Considerations Specific to the Child or Adolescent

Parental oversight is important in the child and adolescent, as there may be younger children in the household, for whom accidental ingestion could be serious or even deadly. Likewise, parents are important for monitoring of opioid use, both for the child and the adolescent, and in that they (the parents) also have access to the opioid themselves. We stress the importance of safekeeping of opioids and other medications with both the patient and the family members.

Peer acceptance is an important part of adolescent and older child socialization. Although internal factors may predispose children or adolescents to increased influence by their peers, social pressure also influences their vulnerability.[21] Thus, the risk of medication misappropriation may be greater in this age group than in adults, not necessarily by intent but potentially by lack of vigilance or even low refusal skills. As we know from studies of adolescent general populations, prescription opioid misuse by those not personally prescribed opioids is higher than in those with opioid prescriptions.[9] The prescription opioid medication necessarily comes from either a prescriber or a person prescribed the drug. The adolescent patient has unique pressures that influence the risk of diversion, both intentional and nonintentional.

School plays an important role in the daily life of the child and adolescent. The school can facilitate pain treatment strategies, to allow both physical and psychological strategies to be integrated into the patient's daily routine. For opioid use, the school may also become intricately involved for monitoring and for distribution of the prescription.

Opioid monitoring is modified for the child or adolescent based on parental involvement in monitoring and in the child's or adolescent's frequent dependence on the caregiver for access to health care providers for monitoring. As such, we use telephone monitoring on a regular basis (weekly at initiation of therapy, and with changes).

Ethical Issues

Despite our continuing efforts to make "children's pain control" a priority, the management of childhood chronic pain can create ethical dilemmas from patient-centered, health care, and societal perspectives.[22,23] Children with chronic pain, like Cassie, depend greatly on their parents (and adult health care providers) to understand, cope, and interpret their pain and its impact on their lives.[24,25] Moreover, parents usually decide (for children) or influence (for adolescents) treatment choices. Health care providers must contend with ethical dilemmas that are inevitably raised when treating child patients, such as:

- Judging benefits, risks, and burdens from the child's and family's perspectives
- Determining children's capacity to understand their pain condition and decide among treatment options
- Resolving disagreements among children and parents as to the "best" treatment regimen, for example, as when Cassie's mom believed that Cassie should use a fentanyl patch

To do so, health care providers are guided by three ethical standards: beneficence (i.e., making decisions to support the child's best interests); informed consent; and the double principle, an action that promotes well-being that may have a foreseen negative effect but in which the good effect outweighs the bad.

Children should be involved in their health care decisions to the greatest extent possible.[26,27] Children usually need a more individualized approach, with concrete age-appropriate examples, to enable them to understand their pain condition and appreciate the benefits and risks of recommended treatments. According to the American Academy of Pediatrics, the dictates of informed consent require that:

1. health care providers use language that is appropriate for a child's developmental age to explain the child's condition, the proposed treatment and associated risks/benefits, and the risks/benefits of alternative treatments (including the choice of no treatment);

2. that children (or parents as surrogate decision makers) have appropriate decision-making capacity, including the ability to understand and communicate information, as well as comprehend the consequences of the proposed treatment, nontreatment, and treatment alternatives; and

3. that children have autonomy, so that to the greatest extent possible, they are free to choose treatment without being coerced or manipulated.[26]

All of this needs to be weighed with the unknown risks of opioid or other substance abuse in children and adolescents and the risk of nonopioid substance abuse in this population. To this end, adolescents who may be capable of consent should be given the opportunity to visit with the health care practitioner independently from parents.

Children need the same care and consideration as their adult counterparts, with the caveat that their caregivers need to be involved in decisions where possible. Greater consideration should be given to the child's or adolescent's ability to understand language used by health care practitioners. And at the same time, there may be less concrete information about long-term consequences of opioid therapy in children and adolescents and of chronic pain, to guide the practitioner and inform the child and his or her family. Likewise, children and adolescents may not be aware of their role in the ethical use of opioids, in that it is their (and their caregivers') responsibility to use medications as prescribed and to keep the medications safe from others, including other household members and friends. Thus, the practitioner should be explicit during discussion regarding the child's and his or her caregivers' role in responsible use of opioids.

Initial Recommendations

Ideally, the prescriber would use opioids only for refractory and well-defined somatic or neuropathic pain that interferes with function or quality of life. Adolescents, as described previously, may be at greater risk for opioid misuse than their older counterparts. As such, assessment of opioid misuse potential is essential for prevention of long-term complications. Nevertheless, it is important to treat pain to help modify the potential for ongoing pain, normalize the patient's social and academic life, and minimize or prevent disability. It would also be important to monitor these patients carefully. In adapting opioid guidelines[28] for this patient population, the following should be considered:

1. Review of personal risk factors

   1.1. Prior alcohol use may not be relevant as the adolescent or child may never have tried alcohol in a significant way. Discussion regarding peer pressure, self-reliance, and family history becomes more important.

2. Overview of potential drug-related side effects and cautions about opioid use

   2.1. Discussion of nonprescription and illicit drugs should be explicit and specific (regarding use of nonprescription drugs in preadolescents and adolescents).

   2.2. Risk of driving during titration of the opioid should be explicitly discussed, as an adolescent's motivation to drive may outweigh his or her concerns for safety.

   2.3. Weight-based calculations of dosing and adult maximum may differ.

   2.4. Discussion of potential but unclear long-term side effects should be included.

   2.5. Discussion of the importance of using medication as prescribed should also be included.

   2.6. Importance of safekeeping of the medication to prevent inadvertent use by another person should be emphasized.

3. Explicit goals of opioid therapy

   3.1. Discussion of outcome expectations should be clear and precise.

      3.1.1. Daily school attendance should be included, perhaps on a modified schedule, developed in collaboration with parents and the school.

      3.1.2. Participation in the recommended physiotherapy and/or pain psychological treatment program should be included.

      3.1.3. Socializing at the previously established level should be included (e.g., out once per week with friends).

      3.1.4. Sustained reduction in pain intensity by a minimum of 30% should be included.

   3.2. Discussion of the plan to stop opioid therapy in the event of failure of the trial should be explicit and clear.

4. Developmental factors

   4.1. Route of administration should be considered for ease of access.

   4.2. Storage method and school/home environment should be considered for safety and ability to administer the opioid as prescribed.

4.3. Language for any opioid agreement should be simplified, to ensure comprehensive understanding (e.g., low-level literacy contract[29]), preferably in a written format.

4.4. Caregivers should be involved in the agreement.

4.5. Opportunity to see the adolescent alone should be provided (e.g., established as a routine for the adolescent).

Initial recommendations for opioid therapy for chronic noncancer pain are based on assessment of the child or adolescent with a complete medical and psychiatric history and physical examination, and failure of other treatments. In keeping with the World Health Organization (WHO) recommendations for mild- to moderate-strength drug treatments, we try acetaminophen and NSAIDs as a first line, where possible. The treatment plan always includes a multidisciplinary approach, introducing the concept of the "3 P's." In other words, treatment includes pharmacotherapy, physical therapy, and psychological therapy. The physical therapy and psychological therapy are ongoing during medication adjustments. The aim is for improvement in children and adolescents with opioid use as part of a multimodal treatment approach.[30] We follow the WHO guidelines for initiating pharmacologic treatment with simple analgesics (such as acetaminophen and/or NSAIDs or cyclooxygenase-2 inhibitors). We supplement simple analgesics with other drugs such as the gabapentinoids or other anticonvulsants, or tricyclic antidepressants/duloxetine where relevant. Prior to initiation of opioids, we commonly try a nonnarcotic with narcotic-type properties or a weak opioid, such as tramadol, either alone or in combination with acetaminophen. This is frequently adequate, but if this fails, a frank and open discussion of the risks and benefits of opioid therapy with the patient and the caregivers then follows. This discussion must include a determination of the goals of therapy, including improvement in both pain scores and function. In Cassie's case, after failure of treatment with gabapentin, amitriptyline, simple analgesics, moderate opioids (tramadol, failed due to nausea unrelieved with ondansetron), and psychological treatments (relaxation and mindfulness) and failure to comply with physiotherapy due to pain, we began the discussion of opioid therapy as an option.

For Cassie, we reviewed her personal risk factors (i.e., alcohol use, illicit drugs, prescription drugs, age of first alcoholic drink, psychiatric history, use of sedative medications, history of sleep apnea). We discussed potential drug-related side effects and cautioned about opioid use (e.g., concurrent consumption of alcohol and street drugs and risk of driving during titration). We reviewed the importance of storage of opioids in a safe location, particularly if there are younger siblings in the home (such as the same location one would use to store a large sum of money). Emphasis was placed on the importance of keeping the prescription for the exclusive use of the child. We also discussed the unknown effects of long-term opioid use in adolescents. We explicitly discussed the goals of therapy, including daily school attendance on a modified schedule (developed in collaboration with her parents and school), participation in a physiotherapy program as recommended, going out with friend(s) once a week for fun and socialization, and a sustained 30% reduction in pain intensity (numerical rating scale), and we documented this using a formal opioid agreement.

Cassie received opioids for a diagnosis of postscoliosis surgery mixed neuropathic/nociceptive pain, after failure of multiple other treatments. She is capable of assisting in the balance of benefits and risks of opioids and therefore is helping to guide treatment. We discussed the plan for the time course of the opioid and the expected treatment outcomes within that time frame.

Long-Term Plan

The plan for opioid maintenance revolves around the initial response to the opioids, following a 6- to 8-week trial. If the dosing is limited by side effects, an opioid rotation should be considered, but once at a reasonable therapeutic level, both side effects and function should be reviewed. The goal is not only for pain relief but also for return to school, social activities, hobbies, and an active lifestyle. If there is no improvement in these areas, this may be considered a treatment failure. This should be followed regularly, with monitoring of the prescriptions and monitoring of the return to function. For Cassie, the opioid agreement contained stipulations including (1) school attendance on a modified schedule, (2) participation in a recommended physiotherapy program, (3) socialization with friends once per week, and (4) a sustained 30% reduction in pain intensity. Follow-up with Cassie resulted in an increase in opioid dosing, but still maintaining the goals of function and 30% reduction in pain scores. Nausea was successfully treated with a nonsedating antiemetic (ondansetron), and the importance of school attendance and participation in physiotherapy was emphasized. Success of treatment should be reviewed on a regular basis and endocrine function monitoring should be considered. For Cassie, although initially the response to opioid resulted in success, this was quite variable. This may be the case, hence the importance of monitoring for change in effect and precise delineation of the goals of therapy at regular intervals.

Summary Points

Health care providers should respectfully ascertain parents' underlying beliefs about opioids and provide concrete information to refute any erroneous beliefs and alleviate unfounded fears—specifically additional information about how chronic pain differs from acute pain, especially its multidimensional aspects and the need for multimodal therapy, and explicit information about the efficacy and risk associated with opioid use.

Health care providers should address any misconceptions and acknowledge parents' dissenting views in a sensitive manner, while maintaining that the primary focus is the best interests of the child. They should also assess the extent to which religious/cultural beliefs may conflict with treatment recommendations and assist families to reach an acceptable solution that is in keeping with their beliefs/values and their child's welfare.

- Start with a comprehensive assessment to ensure opioids are a reasonable choice and to identify risk–benefit balance for the patient.
- Maintain a multimodal management approach to treating the pain.
- Screen for risks of opioid misuse.
- Understand child- and adolescent-specific risks and benefits of short- and long-term opioid use.
- Set effectiveness goals with the patient and inform the patient and the patient's family or caregivers of their role in safe use and monitoring effectiveness.
- Plan and initiate an opioid agreement with the child or adolescent and his or her caregiver(s).
- Initiate with a low dose, increase gradually, and track the dose in morphine equivalents per day—use "watchful dose," 200 mg, as a flag to reassess.[11]
- Watch for any emerging risks/complications to prevent unwanted outcomes including misuse and addiction.
- Stop opioid therapy if it is not effective or risks outweigh benefits.

When looking after child and adolescent patients with chronic pain, a multidisciplinary approach is helpful, particularly when considering the addition of opioids to the treatment plan. Assessment of the patient should encompass school, social, physical, and emotional functioning, as well as pain, and long-term consequences of opioid use should play an important role in determining the appropriateness of their use in pain management. Following the addition of opioids as part of a multimodal (3 P's—pharmacologic, physical, and psychological) approach to pain and special monitoring for both medical and psychosocial complications should be frequent in the adolescent. At this time there are no opioid risk tools available for adolescents. As such, the "one prescriber" rule should be in place. Finally, function is as important as pain relief, especially in the young person. The objective of opioid treatment is to facilitate function while diminishing pain, such that function becomes as close to normal as possible.

References

1. Vuong C, Van Uum SHM, O'Dell L, Lutfy K, Friedman T. The effects of opioids and opioid analogs on animal and human endocrine systems. *Endocrine Rev.* 2010;31(1):98–132.

2. Paturi A, Surani S, Ramar K. Sleep among opioid users. *Postgrad Med.* 2011;123(3):80–87.

3. Ingram SL, Fossum EL, Morgan MM. Behavioral and electrophysiological evidence for opioid tolerance in adolescent rats. *Neuropsychopharmacology.* 2007;32(3):600–606.

4. Boyd CJ, McCabe SE, Cranford JA, Young A. Adolescents' motivations to abuse prescription medications. *Pediatrics.* 2006;118(6):2472–2480.

5. Younger JW, Chu LF, D'Arcy NT, Trott KE, Jastrzab LE, Mackey SC. Prescription opioid analgesics rapidly change the human brain. *Pain.* 2011;152(8):1803–1810.

6. Kennedy B, Panksepp J, Wong J, Krause E, Lahvis G. Age-dependent and strain-dependent influences of morphine on mouse social investigation behavior. *Behav Pharmacol.* 2011;22(2):147–159.

7. Crews F, He J, Hodge C. Adolescent cortical development: a critical period of vulnerability for addiction. *Pharmacol Biochem Behav.* 2007;86(2):189–199.

8. Schneider S, Peters J, Bromberg U, et al. Risk taking and the adolescent reward system: a potential common link to substance abuse. *Am J Psychiatry.* 2012;169(1):39–46.

9. Brands B, Paglia-Boak A, Sproule BA. Nonmedical use of opioid analgesics among Ontario students. *Can Fam Physician.* 2010;56(3):256–262.

10. McCabe SE, Boyd CJ, Cranford JA, Teter CJ. Motives for nonmedical use of prescription opioids among high school seniors in the United States: self-treatment and beyond. *Arch Pediatr Adolesc Med.* 2009;163(8):739–744.

11. Brown SC, Taddio A, McGrath PA. Pharmacological considerations in infants and children. In: Beaulieu P, Lussier D, Porreca F, Dickenson A, eds. *Pharmacology of pain.* Seattle: IASP Press; 2010:529–547.

12. Chambers RA, Taylor JR, Potenza MN. Developmental neurocircuitry of motivation in adolescence: a critical period of addiction vulnerability. *Am J Psychiatry.* 2003;160(6):1041–1052.

13. Paglia-Boak A, Mann RE, Adlaf E, Rehm J. *Drug use among Ontario students, 1977–2009: detailed OSDUHS findings.* (CAMH Research Document Series No. 27). Toronto, ON: Centre for Addiction and Mental Health; 2009.

14. MacGregor R, Evans D, Sugden D, Gaussen T, Levene M. Outcome at 5–6 years of prematurely born children who received morphine as neonates. *Arch Dis Child Fetal Neonat Ed.* 1998;79(1):F40–F43.

15. de Graaf J, van Lingen R, Simons SHP, et al. (2011). Long-term effects of routine morphine infusion in mechanically ventilated neonates on children's functioning: five-year follow-up of a randomized controlled trial. *Pain.* 2011;152(6):1391–1397.

16. Martin BC, Fan MY, Edlund MJ, Devries A, Braden JB, Sullivan MD. Long-term chronic opioid therapy discontinuation rates from the TROUP study. *J Gen Intern Med.* 2011;26(12):1450–1457.

17. Sullivan MD, Edlund MJ, Zhang L, Unutzer J, Wells KB. Association between mental health disorders, problem drug use, and regular prescription opioid use. *Arch Intern Med.* 2006;166(19):2087–2093.

18. Sullivan MD, Ballantyne JC. What are we treating with chronic opioid therapy? *Arch Int Med.* 2012;172(5):433–434.

19. Seal KH, Shi Y, Cohen G, Maguen S, Krebs EE, Neylan TC. Association of mental health disorders with prescription opioids and high-risk opioid use in US veterans of Iraq and Afghanistan. *JAMA.* 2012;307(9):940–947.

20. Ballantyne JC, Sullivan MD, Kolody A. Opioid dependence vs addiction: a distinction without a difference? *Arch Int Med.* 2012;13:1–2.

21. Allen JP, Chango J, Szwedo D, Schad M, Marston, E. Predictors of susceptibility to peer influence regarding substance use in adolescence. *Child Dev.* 2012;83(1):337–350.

22. McGrath PA, Ruskin DA. Ethical challenges for children with chronic pain. In: Schatman ME, ed. *Ethical issues in chronic pain management.* New York: Informa Healthcare; 2007:63–79.

23. McGrath PA, Ruskin DA. Caring for children with chronic pain: ethical considerations. *Pediatr Anesthes.* 2007;17(6):505–508.

24. Craig KD, Lilley CM, Gilbert CA. Social barriers to optimal pain management in infants, children, and adolescents. *Clin J Pain.* 1996;12:232–242.

25. McGrath PA, Dade LA. Strategies to decrease pain and minimize disability. In: Price DD, Bushnell MC, eds. *Psychological methods of pain control: basic science and clinical perspectives, progress in pain research and management.* Vol. 29. Seattle: IASP Press; 2004:73–96.

26. Committee on Bioethics, American Academy of Pediatrics. Informed consent, parental permission, and assent in pediatric practice. *Pediatrics.* 1995;95:314–317.

27. Bioethics Committee, Canadian Pediatric Society. Treatment decisions regarding infants, children and adolescents. *Pediatr Child Health.* 2004;9:99–103.

28. Furlan AD, Reardon R, Weppler C, et al., for the National Opioid Use Guideline Group (NOUGG). Opioids for chronic noncancer pain: a new Canadian practice guideline. *CMAJ.* 2010;182(9):923–930.

29. Wallace LS, Keenum AJ, Roskos SE, McDaniel KS. Development and validation of a low-literacy opioid contract. *J Pain.* 2007;8(10):759–766.

30. Slater M, De Lima J, Campbell K, Lane L, Collins J. Opioids for the management of severe chronic nonmalignant pain in children: a retrospective 1-year practice survey in a children's hospital. *Pain Med.* 2010;11(2):207–214.

Chapter 6

Debilitating Pain

Eija Kalso

The Case

A 60-year-old divorced female patient with multiple health problems is referred to a multidisciplinary pain clinic for a consultation. The patient was diagnosed with SAPHO (synovitis, acne, pustulosis, hyperostosis, osteitis) about 20 years ago. A secondary Sjögren syndrome followed. The patient also has hypertension, hyperlipidemia, type 2 diabetes, and asthma. She suffered several small brain infarctions about 5 years ago and has had cognitive problems ever since. She is also obese, with a body mass index (BMI) of 30.

The patient has had a major pain problem in her anterior chest wall for 15 years and low back pain for 20 years. She has fluctuating pain in several joints. She has had arthroplasty for the right knee. At the moment her worst pain is in her back. The pain radiates to the left leg. In addition, she has pain in her feet and hands. She cannot sleep because of pain. Sjögren disease has caused very dry mucous membranes.

The patient is on extensive medication for her multiple diseases. Her pain is treated with meloxicam 15 mg once a day and two tablets of paracetamol 500 mg plus codeine 30 mg 3 times a day. This medication provides some relief.

List of Considerations

- What are the special features of the underlying conditions that can cause pain (i.e., SAPHO and Sjögren)?
- What pain components does the patient have? How important is inflammation or neuropathy?
- Is rosuvastatin the cause of myalgia?
- Are further examinations needed, for example, magnetic resonance imaging (MRI) for the radiating leg pain? Electroneuromyography (ENMG)?
- Are kidney and liver functions normal?
- Does she take drugs that have relevant interactions with analgesics?
- What is the patient's psychosocial status?
- What is the patient's functional status?

Clinical Discussion

This patient's pain problem consists of nociceptive, inflammatory, and neuropathic pain. Anterior chest wall pain is typical for SAPHO. Up to 65% to 90% of these patients have hyperostosis, sclerosis, and bone hypertrophy involving particularly the sternoclavicular joint. There is often also a soft tissue component. Peripheral arthritis is a common problem, too. Sjögren syndrome with dry mucous membranes, dry mouth, and dry eyes can be a secondary complication.

Treating the underlying diseases should alleviate inflammation, and thus disease-modifying therapies are essential. Corticosteroids have previously provided significant relief. Nonsteroidal anti-inflammatory analgesics have also provided pain relief. However, the patient has high blood pressure, and she has already had brain infarctions. Thus, the nonsteroidal anti-inflammatory drugs pose a high risk to this particular patient. According to the literature, synovitis and osteitis related to SAPHO have been treated with tumor necrosis factor-α antagonists, so this may be one alternative in addition to local steroid injections.

Statins can sometimes cause severe myalgia. This patient did not think starting rosuvastatin increased muscle pain. However, she had had another statin earlier that had caused severe myalgia, which ended when the drug was changed.

The patient has normal kidney and liver function.

The patient has two types of neuropathic or neurogenic pain. The ENMG revealed mild sensory polyneuropathy, which may be related to diabetes. The radiating pain in the left leg could be due to spondylodiscitis, which is prevalent in SAPHO. This was excluded with MRI, which did not indicate any spinal stenosis or nerve root compression either. The main finding was degenerative changes.

The best drug for neuropathic pain in this case should improve sleep in addition to relieving pain and should not cause further weight gain or dryness of the mucous membranes. Tricyclic antidepressants at low doses are the most effective drugs in peripheral neuropathy,[1] and they improve sleep. However, tricyclic antidepressants have anticholinergic effects, which would be particularly undesirable because the patient has very dry mucous membranes. Mirtazapine would be a good choice for sleep problems, but it causes weight gain. It had also already been tried and did not provide any symptom relief. Both gabapentin and pregabalin would be good choices as they have been shown to be effective in neuropathic pain and they improve sleep. Also, they have no known pharmacokinetic interactions, which would be of value in this case as the patient is on several different drugs. Both gabapentin and pregabalin had, however, been tried without beneficial effects. Both of them had caused significant edema and weight gain and no pain relief. Duloxetine has very limited anticholinergic effects and would be a good alternative as it has been shown to be effective in neuropathic pain. Unfortunately, it had also been tried without efficacy. Lamotrigine has not been tried yet. The evidence for its efficacy in neuropathic pain is weak, and it is a challenging drug regarding dose titration to avoid adverse effects.

Tramadol would be a possible choice as it has been shown to be effective in neuropathic pain.[2] It also has a weak opioid effect, which could be beneficial for the nociceptive and inflammatory components of pain. The patient had been on tramadol, but she could not tolerate it because of nausea and vomiting. The combination of paracetamol and codeine helps but does not provide sufficient pain relief. This indicates that the pain might be opioid sensitive. On average, opioids have shown efficacy in nociceptive, inflammatory, and neuropathic pain even though they are not the first-line analgesics in neuropathic pain. Buprenorphine would be the first choice, although in the United States there is not yet much familiarity with this drug for pain treatment. If the patient tolerates it, the dose could be titrated upward and the effects on pain relief recorded.

It is also important to consider other nonpharmacologic therapies. The patient is obese, which makes her joint pain worse. Weight loss would be important. However, she has difficulties with exercising because of her pain. A nutrition therapist might help in planning a diet. Also, a physiotherapist should be consulted to guide the patient in appropriate exercise. Transcutaneous nerve stimulation could be tried.

The patient has not been depressed before. Now she is distressed because a close relative has recently been diagnosed with terminal cancer. A psychologist should be consulted to provide support. Later, relaxation and other pain management techniques could be considered.

Ethical Issues

The patient has several chronic debilitating diseases with different components of pain. The basic principles are to treat her conditions with disease-modifying drugs and with analgesics to provide symptom relief. She has a chronic disease and a life expectancy from several years to a couple of decades. She should remain independent and functional. The ethical principle of alleviating pain and suffering and causing as little harm as possible should be the guiding goal for this patient. If other analgesics cause intolerable adverse effects or have a high risk for serious adverse effects, even though they would be effective (e.g., nonsteroidal anti-inflammatory drugs), stronger opioids should be considered. The ethical principle of not causing more harm than benefit should guide opioid dosing. The pain should be relieved with the opioid in order to be continued. The dose should be titrated according to need when pain escalates and tapered down when pain is less intense following successful treatment of the underlying cause. The physician who has the main responsibility for the patient should follow the treatment and adjust it accordingly.

Initial Recommendations

A physiotherapist is involved and the patient starts a trial with transcutaneous nerve stimulation and a gradual physical exercise program. The patient is referred to a nutrition therapist, upon whose advice the patient starts a diet with a goal of losing weight according to a realistic scheme. The patient is referred to a psychologist for assessment. Participation in a relaxation program is suggested once the patient has recovered from her reactive depression.

Meloxicam is stopped because the patient has several contraindications for its continued use (hypertension, ischemic complications). Lamotrigine is started with slow-dose escalation for neuropathic pain. The combination of paracetamol and codeine is changed to paracetamol 1 g taken 2 or 3 times a day. Buprenorphine is introduced at a low dose first, 0.2 mg 3 to 4 times a day. The dose is increased up to 0.4 mg 4 times a day. If the patient does not tolerate buprenorphine or it does not provide enough pain relief, a slow-release opioid formulation (either morphine or oxycodone) can be started. An appropriate dose should be around 20 to 40 mg of oxycodone or 30 to 60 mg of morphine per day.[3]

The pain clinic also asks for a rheumatologist's consultation regarding the use of disease-modifying drugs (e.g., tumor necrosis factor-α antagonists) and local steroid injections to the joints.

Long-Term Plan

Once the patient's pain is under control, the patient will be referred back to her general practitioner with whom the long-term plan has been negotiated. As the patient tolerated lamotrigine and it relieved neuropathic pain, it can be continued. After initial nausea the patient also tolerated buprenorphine, which provided significant pain relief at the dose of 0.4 mg 3 or 4 times a day. The patient started to sleep better. Her mood also improved.

Buprenorphine can be tapered down once the disease-modifying treatments have improved the patient's condition. It can be started again if the patient's pain exacerbates. It is expected that the patient's pain will continue to fluctuate according to the activity of the underlying condition. Local corticosteroid injections can be considered for synovitis in the hands and ankles. Surgery can also be considered if pain intensifies and does not respond to conservative treatment.

If the patient needs strong opioids (buprenorphine is no longer effective or the pain increases in severity), the general practitioner can start the treatment as the patient has been evaluated at the pain clinic and opioid has been considered a potential alternative. The doses should be kept at a level of 40 to 60 mg of oxycodone or 60 to 90 mg of morphine using slow-release formulations. Rapid-effect formulations such as intranasal or transmucosal fentanyl should not be used in the chronic pain setting because of their abuse liability and reinforcing effect on pain behaviors. Opioid-related adverse effects such as constipation should be actively managed and prevented. Other treatments should be intensified (e.g., the systemic corticosteroid doses increased) in order to allow reduction or stabilization of the opioid dose. The patient may also benefit from short cognitive behavioral therapy to reduce opioid requirement.

A special issue regarding the safety of long-term opioid use in this patient is how the opioid treatment would interfere with the immune system.[4] Both

SAPHO and Sjögren syndrome are autoimmune diseases, and the immune system is critical for disease progression. Opioids can modulate the immune system indirectly through the hypothalamic-pituitary-adrenal (HPA) axis, resulting in the release of glucocorticoids and immunosuppressive hormones. Opioids could thus have similar effects as those anti-inflammatory drugs (e.g., cortisone) that are used to manage autoimmune diseases and inflammation. Opioids can also have a direct interaction on macrophages, T lymphocytes, and NK cells. Whether the effects of opioids have any adverse effects (e.g., increase of infections) has not been answered by the small number of uncontrolled studies conducted so far.

Summary Points

This patient has several diseases and major health concerns. A good multidisciplinary assessment is essential. The general practitioner will be responsible for the coordination of the treatment in the long term. The patient needs help from tertiary care when the symptoms get worse. The rheumatologists and the multidisciplinary pain clinic have an important supportive role. The pain clinic should provide clear instructions to the general practitioner as to how opioid dosing should be done, preferably as interval treatments. The general practitioner should consult the pain clinic if there are any concerns regarding opioid dosing (e.g., dose escalation indicating tolerance).

References

1. Finnerup NB, Sindrup SH, Jensen TS. The evidence for pharmacological treatment of neuropathic pain. *Pain.* 2010;150:573–581.

2. Attal N, Cruccu G, Baron R, Haanpää M, Hansson P, Jensen TS. EFNS guidelines on the pharmacological treatment of neuropathic pain: 2010 revision. *Eur J Neurol* 2010;17:1113–1123.

3. Kalso E, Edwards JE, Moore RA, McQuay HJ. Opioid in chronic non-cancer pain: systematic review of efficacy and safety. *Pain.* 2004;112:372–380.

4. Nonković J, Roy S. Role of the mu-opioid receptor in opioid modulation of immune function. *Amino Acids.* Epub doi:10.1007/s000726-011-1163-0

Chapter 7

Chronic Cancer Pain

Shane Brogan, Perry G. Fine

Severe pain is a common occurrence in cancer, especially patients with solid tumors and those with metastatic disease. Opioids are considered to be a necessary component of cancer pain management, but their use becomes complicated in patients with preexisting pain conditions on chronic opioid therapy or in patients who require high-dose therapy and have long life expectancies. These issues are becoming increasingly prevalent as opioid therapy for chronic noncancer pain has become more widely accepted and as cancer survival has, overall, greatly improved. The case that follows serves to illuminate these complex clinical circumstances, providing an opportunity for preparatory clinical problem solving, in anticipation that oncologists, pain specialists, and palliative care specialists will inevitably and increasingly be responsible for these types of patients' care.

The Case

Tom, a 58-year-old male, has attended our interdisciplinary pain management practice for over 8 years for treatment of neck pain related to osteoarthritis of the cervical spine. He has been adherent to all aspects of his comprehensive treatment plan, including participation in physical and cognitive behavioral therapies. Cervical spine injections were performed with good short-term relief, but Tom did not experience long-term benefit. Multiple medications, including nonsteroidal anti-inflammatory drugs (NSAIDs), muscle relaxants, gabapentin, and topical agents, were tried without improvement in his pain. Tom suffered from significant anxiety that was evaluated and treated by the pain management team psychologist. A psychiatrist had managed his anxiety in the past, using various selective serotonin reuptake inhibitors without significant benefit. Low-dose lorazepam was prescribed as an adjunct for pain and anxiety control, and this effectively abated panic attacks that often were accompanied by severe pain flares.

In the absence of sustained benefit from other therapies, opioids were prescribed. Tom's usual, persistent baseline pain was reasonably well controlled with long-acting opioids, with which he demonstrated no problematic behaviors. Over several years, dose escalation occurred in order to meet functional goals, to the point where he was taking sustained-release oxycodone 80 mg

3 times daily and immediate-release oxycodone 30 mg up to 3 times daily to control incident pain (breakthrough pain) predictably brought on by standing, bending, and walking. Although his function was improved sufficiently to allow him to return to light work on a part-time basis, he continued to report visual analog scale (VAS) pain scores of 6 or greater during follow-up clinic visits.

Several months ago, Tom developed unexplained weight loss and new-onset low back and hip pain. Laboratory and imaging studies revealed that he had advanced prostate cancer with metastatic bony disease to his lower lumbar vertebrae, sacrum, and posterior pelvis. This news created severe anxiety for Tom, which was somewhat reduced when his oncologist told him that with therapy, progression of disease could be markedly slowed; his prognosis for long-term survival was relatively good and measured in years. Notwithstanding this positive news, Tom's pain was now out of control (rated 10/10), and he had been taking his controlled-release oxycodone more than prescribed, up to 6 times per day.

List of Considerations

1. This patient has been on long-term opioid therapy for chronic noncancer pain and now he has a diagnosis of cancer with bone metastases and pain out of control. What are the ramifications with regard to pain management?
2. This patient has been taking more medication than prescribed. How do we interpret this behavior and manage it effectively?
3. Is increasing or rotating his opioids indicated?
4. What are other pain management options?

Clinical Discussion

This patient has been on long-term opioid therapy for chronic noncancer pain and now has a diagnosis of cancer. What are the ramifications with regard to pain management?

It is important at the outset to recognize that Tom presents with a more complex clinical problem than that typically seen in individuals who are "opioid naïve" with similar diagnoses. When patients have been exposed to relatively high doses of opioid analgesics over months to years and then experience a supervening pain disorder (e.g., trauma, surgery, malignancy), pain control can be very challenging. Patients on chronic opioid therapy often have a lower pain tolerance and greater response to a given noxious stimulus (hyperalgesia) and an attenuated or diminished response to opioid analgesics (opioid tolerance).[1,2] The emotional response of getting bad news can also heighten the perception of pain, and so concurrent counseling and appropriate psychopharmacotherapy, if indicated, is an important component of pain management in this type of case. Similarly, coordination of pain management with primary oncologic care (surgical treatment, chemotherapy, radiation therapy) is critically important. Tom may respond well over time to disease-modifying interventions that greatly reduce his pain, but in the interim, he will need aggressive palliation of symptoms.

Because Tom is not responding well to his current dose of controlled-release oxycodone, it is reasonable to consider opioid rotation in addition to adjunctive analgesic therapy (e.g., tricyclic antidepressants, bisphosphonates, calcitonin, corticosteroids) in collaboration with his oncologic treatment team.[3,4] Depending on the cancer care plan, it may be more practical to admit Tom for inpatient management of his pain, which will allow for safer and more efficient medication titration.

This patient has been taking more medication than prescribed. What do I do about this?

First and foremost, it is important to maintain a high-trust relationship, so that patients do not fear abandonment and will be forthcoming, and will accept medication counseling as in their best interest, rather than as punitive or judgmental. Patients need to be educated frankly about the health-related dangers of overusing opioids, especially in combination with benzodiazepines and/or alcohol. Patients who take their opioid medications more than prescribed do so for various reasons, ranging from simple misunderstanding of the prescription details to the compulsive medication use of a patient with an addiction disorder. Between these two extremes are the more common problems of *misuse* (taking medication not as directed, for example, in a desperate attempt to control pain or as self-treatment for anxiety or depression, to induce sleep, to reduce stress, or for positive mood effects—e.g., euphoria, escapism, getting high, etc.). An important differential diagnosis when a patient overuses opioids is the consideration of inadequate dosing relative to the level of pain or impairment due to pain. This phenomenon has been termed "pseudoaddiction," due to the appearance of similar out-of-control behaviors as are typically demonstrated by individuals with frank addiction.[5-7]

Opioid tolerance is an important reason for the development of pseudoaddictive behavior, as patients lose opioid efficacy and try to regain a certain level of perceived analgesia. Furthermore, a lack of patient education, with unrealistic expectations of complete pain relief, can drive patients to consume more medications than prescribed in an effort to attain additional analgesia. Therefore, at the time of initiation of opioid therapy, it is necessary to shape realistic expectations and incorporate nonpharmacologic pain coping strategies. Similarly, if pain intensity increases dramatically, the patient (or caregiver) needs to know who to call and how to obtain help to prevent the maladaptive, but very human, response of taking more medication.

In the chronic cancer pain setting, when pain can escalate quickly due to rapidly advancing pathology, adherence to opioid therapy often is in the opposite direction, with patients underusing their medication and suffering needlessly. Patients will often cite fears about becoming "addicted" or stigmatized as a "drug user" or "weak" or other perceptions of being a failure or "losing the battle" with cancer (e.g., "I don't want my kids to know I'm on this stuff").[8] Others value their cognition over comfort: "I need to be able to drop my kids off to school and do errands; it's hard enough *without* being doped up." Here, the key is careful patient education, reassurance, and meticulous attention to dosing and side effect management.

In this case we have a patient with chronic pain who has now developed new nociceptive foci and has a well-understood reason to report increased pain levels and suffering. While no patient should be commended for self-titration of his or her medications, the circumstances in this case make it unreasonable to treat this individual as if he has committed a major violation of any particular agreement or policy. This is especially so given his previous adherent behavior and historical low risk for substance abuse. Therefore, it would be more appropriate to reevaluate the patient and his response to the increased opioid dose especially because he is already at a very high dose, specifically looking for evidence of improvement and signs of toxicity such as somnolence or hypoventilation.

Once again, this is an important opportunity for education. In the interest of patient safety, it is mandatory to remind patients of the dangers of opioids taken in excess of what they are prescribed and to educate the patient (and family, if applicable) about their safe and responsible use. A careful reevaluation of the pain treatment plan, including the role of opioid therapy, should be undertaken, and thought should be given to more measured dose escalation and/or opioid rotation. If there is suspicion of abuse or diversion (it is naïve to assume cancer cures these traits, but our sense of empathy can blind us to this), the usual precautions should be taken, including urine drug testing and routine queries of your state's prescription database, if available.

Is increasing or rotating his opioids indicated?

Opioid switching is recommended when titration leads to an inadequate therapeutic response or intolerable adverse effects dominate.[9,10] Pitfalls of opioid rotation include difficulty with accurate dose conversion with the attendant risks of under- or overdosage, particularly with higher-dose therapy because established "equianalgesic" conversion guidelines are not empirically tested at high ranges. A common strategy to avoid this is to approximate an equianalgesic dose based on accepted conversion tables and automatically reduce the dose by 25% to 50%, and provide the patient with additional breakthrough medications to use in the event of the dose being insufficient.[10] The choice of drug is based on specific characteristics of the drug (e.g., methadone has potentially beneficial dual opioid and N-methyl-D-aspartate (NMDA) receptor activity, but has potentially toxic QTc interval prolongation properties), a patient's previous experience (i.e., known sensitivities or demonstrated efficacy), preferred route of administration (e.g., oral, transmucosal, transdermal, rectal, parenteral, intrathecal), formulation (e.g., rapid onset, short acting, long acting, tamper resistant/abuse deterrent), cost, and convenience. In Tom's case, several options exist because he has only had experience with oxycodone.

When prescribing long-term opioids for the management of pain, an often overlooked consideration is the predicted duration of therapy. For example, in a 35-year-old with chronic low back pain, can one reasonably expect that opioid therapy is a viable option for the remaining 50 years of his life? Strong consideration must be given to the likelihood that this prolonged duration of therapy will result in numerous sequelae of long-term opioid therapy including tolerance, hormonal derangements, opioid-induced hyperalgesia, and very significant health care costs. On the other end of the life expectancy spectrum, in the patient with imminently terminal disease, these considerations are unimportant compared with the short-term goals of patient comfort and optimizing quality of life with little regard for the doses required to achieve this. In modern oncology, an intermediate time frame is now becoming the norm, with many patients surviving with active disease for years or decades, sustained by surgeries, chemotherapy, and radiotherapy. Pain management during this prolonged course can be challenging, as patients have time to develop opioid tolerance, and vigilance on the part of the pain practitioner is required to keep abreast of disease progression and its clinical presentation. Furthermore, pain will be noted to wax and wane, with improvement in symptoms after disease-modifying interventions that lead to tumor regression, requiring opioid dose reduction.

A subset of cancer patients will be fortunate enough to achieve a prolonged remission ("cure") with little chance of disease recurrence, but they are often significantly impaired by the sequelae of their oncologic therapies. It is quite typical for patients in complete remission to expect to return quickly to their prediagnosis level of functioning, but many are surprised by their physical and cognitive impairments, and euphoric relief at getting good prognostic news can quickly turn to frustration. The prevalence of chronic pain in cancer survivors is not well known, but in a study of breast cancer survivors, 47% reported ongoing pain.[11] In the cancer survivor with chronic pain, the management model will be similar to that used for noncancer pain, but special attention should be given to painful conditions related to cancer treatment, such as chemotherapy-induced painful peripheral neuropathy, postmastectomy syndromes, and postthoracotomy syndromes. In addition, the practitioner needs to be vigilant for evidence of disease recurrence, and new or differing pain complaints should be thoroughly investigated.

What are other pain management options?

For Tom, it is becoming apparent that conventional opioid therapy is failing to achieve satisfactory pain control. This is often the case with severe cancer pain, and so a modification of the conventional World Health Organization 3-Step Ladder has been proposed, including the role of interventional therapies.[12] Due to the extreme suffering attendant to a diagnosis of malignant disease, a broad approach to assessment and management must be undertaken. Pain control can only be effectively achieved when psychic distress is also taken into account and treated.[13] This is not to invalidate physical contributions to the experience of pain, but rather to clinically validate current understanding of pain as an integrative function of consciousness. Therefore, access to professionals who can help understand nonnociceptive inputs into Tom's pain experience is critically important. Meanwhile, concurrent medical management, focusing on both disease-modifying and palliative interventions while evaluating and treating pain, treatment side effects such as bowel and bladder function, and common nonpain symptoms including fatigue and nausea, should be an ongoing focus of overall care.

Consultation with a functional restoration team including physical and occupational therapists; physical medicine and rehabilitation specialists; and prosthetics, speech, ostomy, and nutritional therapists should be obtained when significant physical impairment related to the cancer treatment and its sequelae are noted.[14] Many cancer patients have endured major surgeries resulting in various impairments that severely impact function and self-image and cause chronic pain. Oftentimes, rehabilitation from these insults is overlooked, as the emphasis shifts to chemotherapy and radiation therapy so that cancer remission is optimized. While this modern paradigm is often successful in achieving a reduction in tumor burden, a lengthy remission, or a cure, many patients are left with long-term chronic pain. Even in the absence of obvious physical impairment, it is common for cancer patients to emerge from their prolonged treatments in a deconditioned state, and a physical therapy plan to rehabilitate the patient toward normal function can be very helpful. The graduated return to physical activity not only is therapeutic in the physical sense but also can have a very positive effect on mood and sense of well-being.

In the case of cancer pain where a clear source of nociception is often identified, numerous strategies exist to alleviate pain. Systemic therapy with opioids is the most common means by which this is achieved, but alternative pharmacologic agents should also be considered. A multimodal analgesic approach will often yield superior results and, importantly, can offer an opioid dose-sparing effect. In inflammatory conditions, including bony metastatic disease, NSAIDs should always be considered unless contraindicated. The cyclooxygenase-2 (COX-2) selective variety of NSAIDs does not have any greater analgesic efficacy but may be useful when gastrointestinal tolerability is a concern in the short term, and especially when platelet function needs to be maintained. Drugs used in the treatment of neuropathic pain, such as the gabapentinoid anticonvulsants and the tricyclic antidepressants, should be considered when there is clinical evidence of pain originating from peripheral or central nervous system disease.[15]

When pain is reported in a discrete area, thought should be given to local treatments rather than systemic therapy with its associated toxicities.[16] For example, a single symptomatic bone metastasis may be irradiated with excellent pain relief and minimal risk. An acute vertebral fracture may be successfully palliated with a vertebral augmentation procedure such as vertebroplasty or kyphoplasty.[17] Various nerve block procedures with neurolytic substances can be used to interrupt the nerve supply to an anatomic area. Examples include celiac plexus neurolysis for pancreatic cancer pain, which has 70% to 90% efficacy and an excellent safety profile.[18]

In selected patients, the neuraxial delivery of analgesics can be effective when conventional management has failed or is poorly tolerated due to side effects. Optimal timing of this form of interventional therapy remains controversial. Whereas some pain experts believe that neuraxial opioid delivery should be reserved for patients with limited life expectancy (e.g., less than a year), others have reported positive outcomes over longer periods of time compared to high-dose opioid therapy.[19] A small catheter is placed in the cerebrospinal fluid (CSF) of the intrathecal space, and small quantities of medication (e.g., opioids, local anesthetics, clonidine, the calcium channel blocker ziconotide) are delivered adjacent to the spinal cord and nerve roots, where they adsorb onto receptors and ion channels and mediate pain relief.[20,21] In the case of water-soluble opioids, such as morphine, medication will also diffuse and circulate in the CSF rostrally to the brainstem, where additional opioid receptors are located. Given intrathecally, the potency of opioids is 200 to 300 times greater than the oral route, so better analgesia is usually obtained with much reduced systemic toxicity of alternative routes. Depending on the clinical circumstances, intrathecal drug delivery can be accomplished either using an external pump system or using an implanted, refillable and programmable pump. A randomized controlled trial of comprehensive medical management versus intrathecal drug delivery has shown improved clinical outcomes and a trend toward improved survival in patients with refractory pain who receive intrathecal therapy.[22]

Ethical Issues

Tom is dealing with the diagnosis of a condition that, although not imminently terminal, has significant life-limiting implications.[23] The critical ethical issues to consider are support of his autonomy (self-determination) through the provision of ample time to invite discussion of his values and goals, and to provide information in a way that allows him to make informed decisions about all aspects of care. Patients like Tom, who face dramatic life-altering circumstances, can be easily led down paths of false hope (i.e., "cure," or marginally beneficial treatments at great personal or financial cost). The balance of "doing no harm" (nonmaleficence) and "doing good" (beneficence) is not always as easy to strike as these ethical tenets so starkly dichotomize. But this balance, reflecting the "art" of medicine, can be best realized by creating a relationship that invites open, frank, empathic discussion and that continually evaluates and reevaluates the consequences of decisions. Recognition of one's own limits of knowledge, skill, time, and temperament, as well as seeking consultation from other professionals when patient needs and circumstances dictate, is an ethical imperative that requires conscious and conscientious reflection. It is key that care be coordinated to avoid unnecessary redundancy, excessive cost, and avoidable harms from unwitting drug–drug or drug–disease interactions. Tom's circumstances, as elaborated throughout this discussion, suggest multiple opportunities for coordinated care across disciplines to optimize therapeutic outcomes.

Initial Recommendations

After re-education regarding the safe use of opioids, framed in the spirit of, "We want to help treat your pain more effectively but don't want you to hurt yourself with too much medication," Tom's dose of sustained-release oxy-codone was increased to 160 mg bid, and immediate-release oxycodone 30 mg every 3 to 4 hours PRN was prescribed for breakthrough pain, with a maximum of eight doses per day. The potential benefits and risks of adding an NSAID were discussed. He acknowledged that he was already using occasional over-the-counter ibuprofen 200 mg, and he had never had gastritis or peptic ulcer disease, so he was instructed to increase this to 800 mg tid along with a proton pump inhibitor for gastric protection, with ongoing assessment for response and tolerability

Given his history of anxiety and the likelihood that some of his excessive medication use was in an effort to treat his anxiety symptoms, as well as the fact that he was in the process of adjusting to the reality of a life-threatening illness, Tom reinitiated therapy sessions with our psychologist. In coordination with his oncologist, a radiation oncology consultation was arranged, with consideration for radioisotope therapy given the diffuse spread of his disease.

Long-Term Plan

Tom conscientiously complied with cognitive behavioral treatment by our team psychologist and acknowledged that his anxiety had become more manageable. However, this progress suffered a setback when his wife unexpectedly filed divorce proceedings, but our psychologist was well positioned to help deal with this additional burden as it unfolded.

Oral antiandrogen therapy was prescribed by Tom's oncologist and was tolerated well. A bisphosphonate, zoledronic acid, was administered monthly to promote bone integrity and attenuate pain. External beam and radioisotope radiotherapy was considered to be unlikely to significantly help his symptoms.

Tom's pain continued to be difficult to manage with several different opioid analgesics. He developed significant daytime somnolence that negatively impacted his function. After his oncology team was consulted, an intrathecal pump was implanted and an infusion of hydromorphone and bupivacaine was initiated. He was also given a patient-controlled intrathecal analgesia device (Patient Therapy Manager [PTM] from Medtronic) to help control his incident pain and allow for self-titration of intrathecal dosing. His oral opioid therapy was successfully weaned over several days as his intrathecal dosing was simultaneously increased. Although his short-acting oral opioid (oxycodone immediate release) was also discontinued and he was encouraged to use the PTM for breakthrough pain, he repeatedly asked for "a pill to take when the pain is bad." Realizing that he had been on oxycodone for many years and likely had a psychological dependence on this medication and perhaps used it to allay his anxiety symptoms, it was decided to concede and prescribe him a structured number of doses daily rather than create an adversarial interaction and possibly lose his trust.

Thereafter, with intrathecal hydromorphone 6 mg/day and bupivacaine 30 mg/day, his function improved significantly with improved cognition and energy levels, though he never reported anything less than moderate pain (5/10 on VAS). Tom's outlook has improved markedly and he has developed a practical and constructive approach to the remaining years of life. With the help of his sister, he is presently on a road trip from Utah to Georgia to locate and reunite with their estranged brother.

Summary Points

- Importance of open channels of communication and empathic approach toward understanding the nature of Tom's pain and overall suffering
- Have a "game plan" for structured evaluation and reevaluation of symptoms, patient attainable goals, ongoing monitoring of clinical outcomes, and flexibility of treatment approaches, including multimodal and interventional therapies
- Coordinate care among providers, with a designated "medical home," that is, one individual overseeing care (usually oncologist in cancer care setting); incorporate behavioral/psychological and rehabilitative therapies into overall cancer and pain care
- Respect patient choices after full and clearly articulated elaboration of treatment options and likely outcomes
- Assess and treat both continuous (baseline) and breakthrough pain, in order to minimize adverse effects of pain on quality of life.[24]

References

1. Chang G, Chen L, Mao J. Opioid tolerance and hyperalgesia. *Med Clin North Am.* 2007;91(2):199–211.

2. Chu LF, Angst MS, Clark D. Opioid-induced hyperalgesia in humans: molecular mechanisms and clinical considerations. *Clin J Pain.* 2008;24(6):479–496.

3. Major PP, Lipton A, Berenson J, Hortobagyi G. Oral bisphosphonates: a review of clinical use in patients with bone metastases. *Cancer.* 2000;88(1):6–14.

4. Mercadante S, Fulfaro F. Management of painful bone metastases. *Curr Opin Oncol.* 2007;19(4):308–314.

5. Savage SR, Joranson DE, Covington EC, Schnoll SH, Heit HA, Gilson AM. Definitions related to the medical use of opioids: evolution towards universal agreement. *J Pain Symptom Manage.* 2003;26(1):655–667.

6. Ballantyne JC, LaForge KS. Opioid dependence and addiction during opioid treatment of chronic pain. *Pain.* 2007;129(3):235–255.

7. Lusher J, Elander J, Bevan D, Telfer P, Burton B. Analgesic addiction and pseudo-addiction in painful chronic illness. *Clin J Pain.* 2006;22(3):316–324.

8. Reid CM, Gooberman-Hill R, Hanks GW. Opioid analgesics for cancer pain: symptom control for the living or comfort for the dying? A qualitative study to investigate the factors influencing the decision to accept morphine for pain caused by cancer. *Ann Oncol.* 2008;19(1):44–48.

9. Fine PG, Portenoy RK. Establishing "best practices" for opioid rotation: conclusions of an expert panel. *J Pain Symptom Manage.* 2009;38(3):418–425.

10. Knotkova H, Fine PG, Portenoy RK. Opioid rotation: the science and the limitations of the equianalgesic dose table. *J Pain Symptom Manage.* 2009;38(3):426–439.

11. Gartner R, Jensen MB, Nielsen J, Ewertz M, Kroman N, Kehlet H. Prevalence of and factors associated with persistent pain following breast cancer surgery. *JAMA.* 2009;302(18):1985–1992.

12. Fine PG. The evolving and important role of anesthesiology in palliative care. *Anesth Analg.* 2005;100(1):183–188.

13. Abernethy AP, Keefe FJ, McCrory DC, et al. Behavioral therapies for the management of cancer pain: a systematic review. In: Kalso E, Flor H, Dostrovsky JO, eds. *Proceedings of the 11th World Congress on Pain.* Seattle: IASP Press; 2009:789–798.

14. Fu JB, Shin KY, Gillis TA, *Rehabilitation medicine interventions.* In: Bruera PR, ed. *Cancer pain: assessment and management.* Cambridge University Press; 2010:354–376.

15. Caraceni A, Zecca E, Bonezzi C, et al. Gabapentin for neuropathic cancer pain: a randomized controlled trial from the Gabapentin Cancer Pain Study Group. *J Clin Oncol.* 2004;22(14):2909–2917.

16. Brogan S, Junkins S. Interventional therapies for the management of cancer pain. *J Support Oncol.* 2010;8(2):52–59.

17. Burton AW, Reddy SK, Shah HN, Tremont-Lukats I, Mendel E. Percutaneous vertebroplasty—a technique to treat refractory spinal pain in the setting of advanced metastatic cancer: a case series. *J Pain Symptom Manage.* 2005;30(1):87–95.

18. Eisenberg E, Carr DB, Chalmers TC. Neurolytic celiac plexus block for treatment of cancer pain: a meta-analysis. *Anesth Analg.* 1995;80(2):290–295.

19. Deer T, Krames ES, Hassenbusch SJ, et al. Polyanalgesic consensus conference 2007: recommendations for the management of pain by intrathecal (intraspinal) drug delivery: report of an interdisciplinary expert panel. *Neuromodulation.* 2007;10(4):300–328.

20. Stearns L, Boortz-Marx R, Du Pen S, et al. Intrathecal drug delivery for the management of cancer pain: a multidisciplinary consensus of best clinical practices. *J Support Oncol.* 2005;3(6):399–408.

21. Brogan SE. Intrathecal therapy for the management of cancer pain. *Curr Pain Headache Rep.* 2006;10(4):254–259.

22. Smith TJ, Staats PS, Deer T, et al. Randomized clinical trial of an implantable drug delivery system compared with comprehensive medical management for refractory cancer pain: impact on pain, drug-related toxicity, and survival. *J Clin Oncol.* 2002;20(19):4040–4049.

23. Fine PG. The ethical imperative to relieve pain at life's end. *J Pain Symptom Manage.* 2002;23(4):273–277.

24. Davies AN, Vriens J, Kennett A, McTaggart M. An observational study of oncology patients' utilization of breakthrough pain medication. *J Pain Symptom Manage.* 2008;35(4):406–411.

Chapter 8

Pain After Trauma (Including PTSD)

William C. Becker, Robert D. Kerns

The Case

PFC Juan Gonzales is a 25-year-old, single Hispanic male veteran, admitted to the inpatient psychiatric service at the VA Connecticut Healthcare System after being brought in under police custody. He was driving erratically, was stopped by police, and registered a 0.198 alcohol level by breathalyzer. While in the medical emergency department, he expressed passive suicidal ideation: "with all this pain and nightmares, I sometimes think this would all be gone if I wasn't here anymore." He was subsequently admitted to the psychiatric service for alcohol detoxification and monitoring. Consultation was requested by the pain consult service.

As a result of a blast injury approximately 1 year earlier while deployed in Iraq, PFC Gonzalez has a disc injury with L4-L5 radiculopathy, headache, and posttraumatic stress. He had been ejected from a Humvee after running over an improvised explosive device (IED) and experienced concussive head trauma, acute disc herniation, and extensive abrasion/"road rash" on his face and torso from landing and sliding on the road. He spent 3 weeks at the Balad Army Hospital in Iraq and then was transferred to the Landstuhl Regional Medical Center in Germany for 3 months for a patch skin graft from his left thigh to his face. He was then transferred to Walter Reed Army Medical Center for 4 months of rehabilitation. He had returned home to Connecticut 4 months ago.

PFC Gonzalez had completed a remaining two credits required for graduation from state university while deployed in Iraq (online course material) and was currently living with his parents. He was unemployed and in a 4-year on-again, off-again relationship with a woman he met while in high school. He smokes half a pack of cigarettes per day and reports drinking 2 to 3 times per week up to 12 beers. PFC Gonzalez denied illicit drug use.

He reported taking his medications as prescribed except alprazolam, which he takes sometimes during the day if feeling "jittery." He takes prescribed oxycodone in combination with alcohol frequently.

Current medications are escitalopram 10 mg daily, extended-release oxycodone 180 mg (OxyContin 30 mg, two tablets 3 times daily), immediate-release oxycodone 5 mg with APAP 325 mg one to two tablets every 6 hours as needed for breakthrough pain, gabapentin 300 mg 3 times daily, and alprazolam 0.5 mg PO nightly as needed for insomnia.

List of Considerations

- Treatment of chronic pain in soldiers with posttraumatic stress disorder (PTSD) and head injury resembles management of those civilians exposed to physical and psychological violence.
- A multimodal plan of care is needed during transition from acute to chronic pain, assessing multisystem medical and psychosocial factors.
- Shared decision making should improve treatment engagement and outcomes.

Clinical Discussion

PFC Gonzalez's case presentation is complex and, unfortunately, increasingly common. The triad of PTSD, mild traumatic brain injury (mTBI), and chronic pain was found to be more common than any of the three disorders alone in returning Operation Enduring Freedom/Operation Iraqi Freedom (OEF/OIF) soldiers.[1,2] Though this case focuses on a soldier, we know that violence and trauma, both physical and psychological, are also prevalent in the US civilian population and can predispose individuals to a similar clinical picture.[3]

For this patient in particular, and in patients with chronic pain after trauma in general, the emerging data suggest that aggressive pain control may decrease the likelihood of central sensitization and other maladaptive biologic phenomena that contribute to chronic pain.[4] There is a need for providers and patients to be especially cognizant of the transition from acute care posttrauma. Whereas a biomedical approach to chronic disease management has historically been the standard, a biopsychosocial approach is more appropriate here. This distinction has wide-ranging implications for our care of patients with chronic pain following trauma, from how we communicate with patients to the expectations and goals of care to the treatments we offer and the systems of care we design.[5,6] There is a crucial role for a broad yet detailed biopsychosocial assessment to understand an individual's treatment needs as well as the co-occurring conditions that may alter the clinical approach.[7] For treatment of chronic pain after trauma to be successful, it must employ a multimodal plan of care that addresses the multisystem nature of chronic disease.[2] A last consideration is the movement toward patient-centered assessment and treatment: soliciting the patient's input and preferences and incorporating a shared decision-making approach. Ideally, this will improve the likelihood that the patient will engage in treatment.[8,9]

Aggressive treatment of pain posttrauma is becoming increasingly recognized not only as an ethical requirement to reduce needless suffering but also as potentially protective of the development of central sensitization and other phenomena associated with chronic widespread pain.[4,5] Survival rates of wounded soldiers have increased since the Vietnam era,[10] thanks in part to more rapid transport to higher levels of care. PFC Gonzalez had been airlifted to Landstuhl Regional Medical Center in Germany, a state-of-the-art military hospital where his acute injuries were aggressively managed, and was then transitioned successfully to subacute rehabilitation treatment at the Walter Reed Army Medical Center.

PFC Gonzalez's care became more fragmented and, as a result, less effective with his transition from acute to chronic disease management, coinciding with his discharge from active military duty. This is not a unique problem; the US health care system as a whole has been summarily criticized for its focus on acute care with few incentives to promote chronic disease management. The Veterans Health Administration (VHA) and other progressive health care systems are increasingly aware that to improve outcomes in chronic diseases such as chronic pain, care has to be managed: Patients must be actively recruited into care, engaged with interdisciplinary teams, and tracked longitudinally to remain involved with an active plan of care. Nonetheless, it seems as if the patient in this case may have fallen through the cracks.

Several features of this case illustrate the importance of a broad yet detailed biopsychosocial assessment. It is likely that PFC Gonzalez has several co-occurring conditions—chronic pain, major depression, PTSD, alcohol abuse—that will each require treatment to lead to a successful overall outcome. Furthermore, awareness of these co-occurring conditions should help his providers more carefully consider the appropriateness of individual components of his treatment. For example, with a known history of mTBI, an assessment of ongoing cognitive limitations is needed to understand how to structure vocational training, medication regimens, and follow-up. Furthermore, in addition to cognitive function, a comprehensive psychosocial functional assessment is needed including social support; intrapersonal dynamics; coping skills; insight, values, and beliefs related to pain and suffering; and treatment goals and expectations.

As evidenced in even this brief vignette, PFC Gonzalez's combination of PTSD, chronic pain, mTBI with potential cognitive dysfunction, major depression, and alcohol abuse affects quality of life and functioning in multiple domains. As such, multimodal care involving behavioral treatment, pharmacologic therapies, and rehabilitation services was the starting point for any discussion of his treatment. Often the question arises, is there a recommended place to start? Or, should some modalities versus others be favored in the beginning of treatment? Certainly, for each individual patient and his or her clinical circumstances, there will be modalities that may take a more central role and there will be more acute conditions that will deserve attention first. The discussion to follow of specific recommendations for this patient will highlight these considerations.

Sole reliance on opioid analgesics as treatment in a complex case such as this is not a plan that any thoughtful provider would endorse prospectively, but this can sometimes result when the patient is not following through with other treatment modalities or referrals. Such an outcome—sole reliance on opioids—may indicate a developing substance use disorder, but at the very least, it is unlikely to produce a satisfactory outcome for the patient or the provider. It is incumbent on the provider to be vigilant for compliance with all aspects of treatment and insist on multimodal care as a necessary condition for continued opioid therapy. Recently published clinical practice guidelines for chronic opioid therapy are key resources for guiding rationale use of opioids for management of complex chronic pain and associated comorbidities such as those represented by this case.[11,12]

PFC Gonzalez is the case of a soldier who, up until this point in his young life, had been healthy, capable, and in control but is now compromised and in crisis; this is a strong illustration of a broader tenet of chronic pain care: To engage him, the approach to treatment must be patient centered. Communication must be clear and in language he can understand, without jargon. Rationale for treatment must be transparent and explained thoroughly, again in terms that are readily understandable. Where possible, he should be presented with choices; the patient's preferences in these choices should hold the most weight. Family members and other supportive people in the patient's life should also be engaged, but only if the patient makes it clear that this is acceptable. Overall, the patient must be afforded some degree of control to keep him working in a positive, self-efficacious manner.

Ethical Issues

Several ethical questions may arise regarding chronic pain after trauma. One is a broad question that could be applied to a wide range of clinical scenarios: How does a provider deal with the clinical uncertainty related to the potential harm and benefits of opioids? For example, in this case, we have a patient with multiple risk factors for misuse of opioids: young age, active substance abuse, and mental health disorders. These are all purported risk factors for unintentional opioid overdose, although, in fact, these risks are based on inferences from observational studies from which, strictly speaking, causation cannot be determined. Lacking is a clear-cut measure analogous to the international normalized ratio (INR) measurement for warfarin therapy, where prospective data exist showing that risk for well-defined outcomes is elevated either below or above the target level.

At one end of the spectrum, a provider might simply present the potential harms and benefits, acknowledging the limitations of what is known about respective probabilities, and allow the patient to decide which treatment option to pursue. This model weighs patient autonomy heavily but ignores the issue that at least some patients' desire to take opioids is related to opioids' reward-reinforcing pharmacologic properties. On the other hand, a provider may take the stance that opioids are too high risk for a certain patient and not even offer them as an option. This paternalistic approach relies heavily on providers' judgment of what constitutes elevated risk, a calculation that may be fraught with bias, error, and unfairness. Another related ethical quandary is whether and to what degree providers should consider the potential long-term deleterious effects of opioids—including hypogonadism, osteoporosis, hyperalgesia, physical dependence, and addiction—when determining whether opioids should be continued, especially, as in this case, when the patient is young and has the potential for decades of exposure.

Though expert guidelines do not address these ethical dilemmas per se, a recommended approach can be extrapolated. Providers should be aware of those factors representing best evidence for elevated risk of harm from opioid therapy and then select patients for therapy based on determination of whether potential benefit is likely to outweigh harm.[11,12] This assessment should be thorough and as standardized as possible to maintain a consistent process.

Initial Recommendations

For PFC Gonzalez, initial recommendations for management were wide-ranging. Here was a patient in crisis—a young man with co-occurring major depression, chronic pain, PTSD, substance abuse, and possible cognitive deficits who had expressed passive suicidal ideation. The urgent goal of care was that he immediately be kept safe from harming himself; other goals of care remained secondary until that risk was deemed negligible.

While an in-patient, PFC Gonzalez stabilized from the standpoint of acute suicidal risk. He underwent a comprehensive assessment of his functional status across a wide variety of domains. A neuropsychological evaluation assessed cognitive function and made definitive diagnoses regarding mood, thought, and personality disorders. He was formally assessed for the presence of substance use disorders using the Composite International Diagnostic Interview—Substance Abuse Module (CIDI-SAM); readiness to change regarding hazardous drinking/alcohol abuse is a separate key component to the substance abuse assessment. Physical and occupational therapists as well as vocational rehabilitation specialists evaluated his limitations in each of these areas. A generalist competent in pain assessment updated a careful, detailed pain history and general physical examination and reevaluated diagnostic workup regarding the pain-generating disease processes, determining that knee x-rays to assess presence and/or degree of early osteoarthritis were not needed and that magnetic resonance imaging (MRI) of the L-spine was not necessary because no focal neurologic deficits were found on his physical examination.

In PFC Gonzalez, as in others, specific treatment recommendations depended on the results of these assessments, but generally speaking, recommendations would follow the multimodal paradigm. Cognitive processing therapy and prolonged exposure (PE) therapy are two evidence-based behavioral interventions for PTSD that should be considered, possibly in conjunction with targeted pharmacotherapy, likely a selective serotonin reuptake inhibitor (SSRI).[13] A novel approach to provide integrative psychological treatment for comorbid chronic pain and PTSD has preliminary empirical support and could be considered.[14] As in the present case, therapists are advised to tailor psychological treatment to accommodate patients' cognitive deficits that affect learning.[15] As nightmares are a prominent feature of his symptomatology, prazosin was considered as adjunctive treatment.[16]

Motivational enhancement techniques to move PFC Gonzalez forward in the readiness-to-change spectrum (from precontemplative to contemplative, for example) were employed on a recurring basis.[17] Because he agreed to participate in the mutual-help group Alcoholics Anonymous, his substance use disorder did not appear to require further inpatient intensive rehabilitation. Data on the benefits of adjunctive pharmacotherapies to maintain sustained remission in alcohol use disorders are emerging.

PFC Gonzalez received necessarily wide-ranging pain treatment recommendations.[18] First, he was educated on the specific diagnoses causing pain and their likely prognoses, with special emphasis placed on the notion that disease management including proper back hygiene, self-care techniques, regular exercise, and physical therapy were the only ways to regain function. This psychoeducational approach should always be considered part of all multimodal treatment programs and must be frequently revisited. Next, we suggested targeted pharmacotherapy for nociceptive pain, neuropathic pain, and inflammation, because all three were present in this patient with disc herniation and radiculitis. For nociceptive pain, nonsteroidal anti-inflammatory medications, acetaminophen, and/or opioids were the main options. For neuropathic pain, anticonvulsants, serotonin-norepinephrine reuptake inhibitors, and tricyclic antidepressants are all reasonable options. He was already prescribed gabapentin, which was titrated up over the span of a few weeks to a target dose of 900 mg tid, being mindful of side effects and the potential for sedating interactions with his other medications.

The role of opioids in this case is complex. The first consideration must always be the patient's safety, and using opioids while binge drinking is clearly not safe. However, because PFC Gonzalez had forced abstinence from alcohol while he was an inpatient, restarting opioids during the admission and continuing them postdischarge was trialed. Short courses of medication were started (e.g., 2 to 5 days) with very close follow-up to assess his safe medication-taking practices. He demonstrated safe and effective use of opioids, and so the follow-up interval was increased. Critical to this approach is that informed consent for opioid treatment was obtained from the patient. Furthermore, a discussion between the prescriber and PFC Gonzalez took place regarding the necessity of participating in multimodal care and a checklist of the practice's expectations for his safe medication-taking practices. Whether or not a formal treatment agreement signed by the prescriber and patient is used, this discussion must take place and must be documented. The prescriber must be prepared to discontinue opioid therapy if evident harm to the patient is outweighing benefit.

At each step in this process, a patient-centered approach was employed, including the necessary adjustments to the complexity of the regimen for his diagnosed cognitive deficits. Whenever possible, providers engaged the patient in shared decision making in which both provider and patient discussed their preferences and the rationale for those preferences. This process of transparency and collaboration has been demonstrated to improve both patient and provider satisfaction with treatment.[8,9]

Long-Term Plan

The long-term plan for PFC Gonzalez is to continue to promote engagement with a multimodal plan of care. As rehabilitation progresses and he transitions from acute crisis care to chronic disease management to, ideally, maintenance of high-quality-of-life functional status, his treatment plans will include vocational rehabilitation and employment and relationship counseling to enable him to work toward a fulfilling adult life. Ideally, he will have a longitudinal relationship with a primary care team—the so-called patient-centered medical home—so that robust, integrated care between behavioral health, addiction treatment, and primary and specialty care can be maintained throughout the life cycle.

Summary Points

- Chronic pain after trauma is increasingly prevalent.
- The transition from acute care following trauma to chronic disease management must be an active one to avoid patients disengaging with treatment.
- Epidemiologic data reveal that co-occurring psychological distress, chronic pain, and other conditions are more common than chronic pain in isolation; therefore, a careful assessment to uncover underlying conditions is vital.
- The multisystem nature of chronic pain, especially chronic pain following trauma, dictates a multimodal treatment approach.
- To improve effectiveness, treatment must be patient centered.

References

1. Lew HL, Otis JD, Tun C, Kerns RD, Clark ME, Cifu DX. Prevalence of chronic pain, posttraumatic stress disorder, and post-concussive syndrome in OEF/OIF veterans: the polytrauma clinical triad. *J Rehabil Res Dev.* 2009;46:697–702.

2. Walker RL, Clark ME, Sanders SH. The "postdeployment multi-symptom disorder": an emerging syndrome in need of a new treatment paradigm. *Psychol Serv.* 2010;7:136–147.

3. Phifer J, Skelton K, Weiss T, et al. Pain symptomatology and pain medication use in civilian PTSD. *Pain.* 2011;152(10):2233–2240.

4. Buckenmaier CC 3rd, Brandon-Edwards H, Borden D Jr, Wright J. Treating pain on the battlefield: a warrior's perspective. *Curr Pain Headache Rep.* 2010;14(1):1–7.

5. Aldington D, Kerns RD. Battlefield to bedside to recovery. In: Ballantyne J, ed. *Pain: clinical updates;.* IASP Press; 2011;19(5):1–6.

6. Gallagher RM, Polomano R. Early, continuous, and restorative pain management in injured soldiers: the challenge ahead. *Pain Med.* 2006;7(4):284–286.

7. Gatchel RJ, Peng YB, Fuchs PN, Peters ML, Turk DC. The biopsychosocial approach to chronic pain: scientific advances and future directions. *Psychol Bull.* 2007;133:581–607.

8. Frantsve L, Kerns RD. Patient-provider interactions in the management of chronic pain: current findings within the context of shared medical decision-making. *Pain Med.* 2007;8:25–35.

9. Sullivan MD, Leigh J, Gaster B. Brief report: training internists in shared decision making about chronic opioid treatment for noncancer pain [see comment]. *J Gen Intern Med.* 2006;21(4):360–362.

10. Gawande A. Casualties of war—military care for the wounded from Iraq and Afghanistan. *N Engl J Med.* 2004;351(24):2471–2475.

11. Chou R, Fanciullo GJ, Fine PG, et al. Clinical guidelines for the use of chronic opioid therapy in chronic noncancer pain. *J Pain.* 2009;10(2):113–130.

12. Veterans Health Administration. *VA-DoD clinical practice guideline for the management of opioid therapy for chronic pain.* Washington, DC: Department of Veterans Affairs; 2010. http://www.healthquality.va.gov/COT_312_Full-er.pdf

13. Veterans Health Administration. *VA-DoD clinical practice guideline on managing post traumatic stress.* Washington, DC: Department of Veterans Affairs; 2010. http://www.healthquality.va.gov/PTSD-FULL-2010c.pdf

14. Otis JD, Keane T, Kerns RD, Monson C, Scioli E. The development of an integrated treatment for veterans with comorbid chronic pain and posttraumatic stress disorder. *Pain Med.* 2009;10:1300–1311.

15. Otis JD, McGlinchey R, Vasterling JJ, Kerns RD. Complicating factors associated with mild traumatic brain injury: impact on pain and posttraumatic stress disorder treatment. *J Clin Psychol Med Sett.* 2011;18(2):145–154.

16. Raskind MA, Peskind ER, Hoff DJ, et al. A parallel group placebo controlled study of prazosin for trauma nightmares and sleep disturbances in combat veterans with post-traumatic stress disorder. *Biol Psychiatry* 2007;61:928–934.

17. Miller WR, Rollnick S. *Motivational interviewing: preparing people for change.* 2nd ed. New York: Guilford Press; 2002.

18. Chou R, Qaseem A, Snow V. Diagnosis and treatment of low back pain: a joint clinical practice guideline from the American College of Physicians and the American Pain Society. *Ann Intern Med.* 2007;147:478–491.

Chapter 9

Opioid Therapy in Chronic Painful Disease

Daniel Krashin, Andrea M. Trescot

The Case

Mr. N is a 36-year-old white male, HIV-positive, former IV drug abuser, who has supported himself for many years working as a waiter. His HIV is well controlled with zidovudine, emtricitabine-tenofovir, and etravirine, with which he is very compliant. He has been "clean and sober" for 5 years. He suffers from chronic peripheral neuropathy, which is bilateral and progressive. He has tried physical therapy, along with gabapentin and tramadol, with limited relief. He has been treated with methadone 30 mg/day for this pain by his primary care provider, who also prescribes his HIV regimen; however, this physician has become uncomfortable with continuing methadone due to concerns regarding recent reports of deaths from methadone as well as the patient seeking early refills on more than one occasion. When informed that he may be taken off methadone, the patient becomes visibly upset and states that he would not feel life is worth living if he could not get adequate pain relief. Mr. N has been given a referral to the pain clinic, with only enough medication to get him to this appointment.

List of Considerations

- Opioids in patients with history of substance abuse
- HIV/AIDS and drug–drug interactions
- Neuropathy management

Clinical Discussion

Pain is a common problem among patients infected with HIV, affecting 30% to 67% of these individuals.[1] Koeppe et al.[2] conducted a cross-sectional study of pain in their HIV clinic and found that, despite aggressive attempts at pain management, many patients continued to experience significant pain. Pain can affect people with HIV during the course of their illness, with more severe disease and poor health being associated with more pain and more use of medical care for pain.[3] In addition, the patients with HIV who had comorbid substance abuse issues often had increased pain symptoms.[4]

Opioids in Patients With History of Substance Abuse

Although this topic is covered extensively in Chapter 2, a brief discussion of the issues regarding opioid use in patients with a history of substance abuse disorder (SUD) is pertinent. The use of opioids for pain has been increasing over the last few years; in 2002, reports showed a 222% increase in the absolute number of prescriptions for opioids over the previous 10-year period.[5] One of the most feared complications of opioid therapy is addiction; addiction is composed of four core elements (the 4 C's): **compulsive** use, inability to **control** the quantity used, **craving** the psychological drug effects, and **continued** use of the drug despite its adverse effects.[5] Although the risk of iatrogenic addiction (addiction arising as a direct consequence of opioid pain treatment) is relatively small,[6] this risk appears to be increased in patients with a personal history or family history of substance abuse. In a study of primary care patients treated with opioids for pain, the most frequent behaviors suggestive of addiction included early refills (41.7%), increasing dose without physician consent (35.7%), and feeling intoxicated from opioids (32.2%). Only 1.1% of patients with one to three of these aberrant behaviors (N = 464; 51.2%) met *Diagnostic and Statistical Manual of Mental Disorders*, fourth edition (DSM-IV) criteria for current opioid dependence compared with 9.9% of patients with four or more behaviors (N = 264; 29.3%).[6] In a pain management program within a US academic general internal medical practice, opioid misuse was identified in 32% of patients, with the best predictors of misuse occurring in those patients with a self-reported history of alcohol or cocaine abuse, previous criminal convictions for driving under the influence (DUI), or drug offenses.[7] Aberrancy included urine drug screens positive for stimulants (usually cocaine), repeatedly negative urine screens for prescribed opioids and positive for nonprescribed opioids, regular acquisition of opioids from multiple providers, and forged prescriptions. Primary care providers have justifiable concerns when prescribing opioids to this population, because the overall prevalence of substance use disorders among chronic pain patients is estimated to be between 3% and 18%.[8] The issue is balancing benefit with risk, which of course requires ongoing careful assessments of both.

Special precautions that can be taken for known substance abusers or for individuals at risk include the following:

- Use of opioid agreements or alternative tools to educate patients about drug dangers and responsible drug use
- Special monitoring (pill counts, urine drug screens)
- Monthly follow-up and prescription pick-up

- Mandatory counseling
- Use of single prescribers and pharmacists wherever possible

In some states, prescription-monitoring programs are operating, although not always with physician (as distinct from law enforcement) access. Experts and society guidelines have suggested that long-acting (controlled-release or sustained-release) opioids (LAOs) are useful for patients with continuous pain, whereas short-acting (immediate-release) opioids are used to manage intermittent and breakthrough pain.[9] Because the peak effect of LAOs has a slower onset and lower peak, LAOs are felt to decrease the "pop a pill/feel better" effect seen with short-acting opioids. It has often been suggested that round-the-clock dosing of LAOs improves analgesia and helps control addiction, but a recent epidemiologic study brings these suppositions into question.[10]

Patients who either have or are at risk for sleep apnea also pose special considerations when prescribing any long-acting opioid, so this may be an appropriate screening study for selected patients.[11] The options for LAOs are limited: Tramadol, a weak opioid, is available in a long-acting formulation. Morphine, hydromorphone, oxycodone, and oxymorphone are also available in special formulations to provide a delayed onset/prolonged effect. Fentanyl is available as a time-released patch; buprenorphine has been available as a patch in Europe for many years but has only recently become available in this formulation in the United States. Methadone and levorphanol are inherently long lasting. Methadone has been used most often for the treatment of both SUD and chronic pain; besides being long acting, it also has an inhibitory effect at the N-methyl-D-aspartate (NMDA) receptor, which allows it to provide significant relief for neuropathic pain. It is also very inexpensive, an important issue for patients without insurance coverage.

Drug–Drug Interactions

Highly active antiretroviral treatment (HAART) therapy has revolutionized the treatment of HIV infections; however, it has also introduced a host of new complications to the medical management of these patients. Antiretroviral (ARV) medication may require complex regimens of multiple drugs per day, and there are numerous and complex interactions between the ARV medications themselves and other medications, including pain medications.

Drug–drug interactions with ARV medications may result in decreased blood levels of the ARV medications (resulting in treatment failure), while interactions with pain medicines may lower the effective dose (leaving the patient in pain) or increase the blood levels of the pain medications (risking catastrophic side effects).[12]

Opioids are medications that have their action at the opioid receptors in the brain. The *opiates*, pain medicines *directly* extracted from opium, which include morphine and codeine, are unlikely to cause interactions with ARV medications. Heroin is converted by esterases in the plasma to morphine, and both morphine and codeine are metabolized by glucuronidation. Nelfinavir and

:uronidation, accelerating morphine metabolism, de-
e, and increasing levels of the less pharmacologically
ιnide (M6G) and the potentially hyperalgic morphine-

h are generally metabolized using the P450 enzyme
of drug–drug interactions. For example, oxycodone,
nonsteroidal anti-inflammatory drugs (NSAIDs) or
in long-acting formulations such as OxyContin®, is
to a variety of metabolites, including oxymorphone,
which is about 50% more potent.[15] Consequently, its effective blood level
may change when a CYP2D6 inhibitor such as ritonavir is added or stopped.
Hydrocodone, also commonly used for pain, is metabolized by both CYP2D6
and CYP3A4.[14] Because the action of CYP2D6 is to convert hydrocodone into
the more potent hydromorphone, inhibition of this enzyme will decrease the
overall effect of hydrocodone and may provoke withdrawal symptoms.

Tramadol is a synthetic analog of codeine.[16] The M1 derivative (O-dimethyl
tramadol) produced by CYP2D6 has as much as 6 times higher activity than
the parent compound. Excretion of tramadol is also via CYP2D6. Toxic doses
cause central nervous system (CNS) excitation and seizures, so that CYP2D6
inhibition by ritonavir has the potential for both decreased analgesia and increased toxicity.

Methadone is commonly used as a long-acting pain medication for chronic
pain and also has a role in treatment of opioid dependence. It is a long-acting
mu-opioid receptor agonist, as well as an NMDA inhibitor. Methadone is
metabolized via CYP3A4, CYP2B6, and CYP2C19 with possible activity as
well from CYP4A4. Methadone levels can be influenced by numerous ARVs,
particularly those in the non-nucleoside reverse-transcriptase inhibitor (non-
NRTI) class. Efavirenz and nevirapine can reduce the area under curve (AUC)
for methadone by over 50%, resulting in acute opioid withdrawal and the need
for increased dosing.[17] Etravirine causes a measurable decrease in methadone
activity that is not usually clinically significant.[18]

Protease inhibitor (PI) ARVs are known to act as inhibitors of CYP3A4
in vitro but have been found to decrease methadone levels in vivo.[19] The
combinations of lopinavir/ritonavir and darunavir/ritonavir have been shown to
significantly reduce the AUC of methadone and cause withdrawal symptoms.[19]
As this response is not totally predictable, and as it usually takes 2 to 3 weeks to
manifest, because P450 enzymes must be synthesized, it is usually recommended
to wait several weeks before changing dosing of methadone. However, if these
agents are stopped suddenly, the patient is at risk of overdose with methadone,
because blood levels may rise precipitously.[20]

Methadone can also affect blood levels of some old ARVs, such as
didanosine and stavudine,[21] by impairing absorption through the gastrointestinal tract, and zidovudine by inhibiting its glucuronidation, causing possible
toxicity.[22]

Because methadone is also associated with prolongation of the QTc interval
and at high doses with torsades de pointes, possibly potentiating this same

effect seen with other drugs, such as antidepressant medications, antiarrhythmics, chloroquine, quinolone, macrolide antibiotics, and some antifungals, several experts recommend that pretreatment and possibly periodic cardiograms be obtained in patients using high doses.[23,24]

Buprenorphine is a mu-opioid partial agonist with strong affinity for opioid receptors. It has been used for acute pain for many years and more recently has been used as well for treatment of opioid dependence. It is metabolized via CYP3A4 to an active metabolite and also by CYP2C8. Both the drug and its metabolite are also metabolized by glucuronidation, which reduces the risk of clinically significant medication interaction.[17] Thus, ARVs have so far shown much less risk of interaction with buprenorphine. Efavirenz has been shown to decrease the AUC of buprenorphine, but this has not been clinically significant. However, the PI atazanavir has been shown to increase the AUC of buprenorphine by over 90%, causing significant drowsiness and confusion.[25]

Chronic pain patients will generally be started on long-acting opioids for their pain. Prior to the first prescription, ground rules for pain treatment and a pain agreement should be established. Some patients will have difficulty tolerating a slow titration of long-acting opioid, as there may be a period of inadequate pain relief. Short-acting opioids may be used to help cover this pain temporarily or to treat acute pain exacerbations. This short-acting medication may be of the same medication, as in the case of oxycodone or morphine (which have both short-acting and long-acting formulations), or different, as in the case of methadone (which has no short-acting form). It has been clinically suggested that meperidine and propoxyphene be avoided in this case, as both have short activity, limited analgesic effect, and toxic metabolites [26] Mixed agonist–antagonist opioids such as buprenorphine, nalbuphine, or pentazocine are likely to provoke withdrawal symptoms and render the long-acting opioid medication ineffective.

Patients with a past history of opioid use may need larger doses of opioids to treat pain, as they often have increased tolerance, even if currently abstinent.[27,28] It is important to note that it is illegal under current law in the United States to treat someone for opioid addiction with opioids unless they are properly enrolled with a methadone clinic or Suboxone® prescriber; however, there is no legal restriction on treating legitimate *pain* with opioids, regardless of addiction history.

Methadone is an effective treatment for acute pain and also, due to its long activity time, will help prevent acute withdrawal without producing excessive euphoria. However, as the effective duration of analgesic effect is only 6 to 8 hours, which is less than the half-life of 12 to 16 hours (perhaps even as high as 130 hours),[29] prescribers must be wary of accumulating methadone levels and sedation. In some cases, additional shorter-acting opioids may be necessary to achieve adequate pain control. Most overdoses with methadone occur during the initiation of methadone treatment, indicating that a very slow and carefully observed dose titration for all clinical settings introducing methadone is necessary.[30]

The tricyclic antidepressants bind a wide variety of neurotransmitter receptors and have the potential to affect many more indirectly. Kappa-opioid receptor binding has been found to be inhibited by antidepressants including amitriptyline, nortriptyline, and clomipramine.[31] Tricyclic antidepressants, as well as morphine, are substrates of the uridine diphosphate glucuronyl transferase (UDPGT) enzyme and have the potential to inhibit the glucuronidation of morphine.[31] The clinical significance of this is unclear.

The primary P450 enzymes responsible for tricyclic antidepressant metabolism include CYP1A2, CYP2C19, CYP2D6, and CYP3A3/4 (see Table 9.1).

Table 9.1 Tricyclic Antidepressants and Opioids Metabolized by the CYP P450 Isozymes

P450 Isozyme	Substrates	Inhibitors
CYP1A2	Amitriptyline Clomipramine Imipramine Doxepin	Fluvoxamine Quinolone antibiotics
CYP2B6 CYP2C9	Methadone Warfarin	
CYP2C19	Amitriptyline Clomipramine Imipramine Doxepin	Fluvoxamine (high potential) Fluoxetine (moderate potential)
CYP2D6	Secondary TCAs Dextromethorphan (O-demethylation) Codeine Tramadol	Secondary TCAs (mild/moderate) Quinidine Fluoxetine Norfluoxetine Doxepin Methadone
CYP3A3/4	Amitriptyline Clomipramine Imipramine Doxepin Methadone Dextromethorphan (N-demethylation) Buprenorphine	Norfluoxetine Nefazodone Ketoconazole Other imidazole antibiotics Erythromycin Other macrolide antibiotics Grapefruit juice (bergamottin) Cyclosporine

Abbreviations: TCAs, tricyclic antidepressants.

Notes: Secondary TCAs: desipramine, nortriptyline, and protriptyline.

Tertiary TCAs: amitriptyline, clomipramine, trimipramine, imipramine, and doxepin.

Amitriptyline inhibits the metabolism of both CYP2D6 and CYP3A4, which could lead to increased plasma levels of methadone, although this has not been reported clinically.[32] Methadone also is an inhibitor of CYP2D6 and has considerable variation in plasma levels due to variation of enzymatic activity.[29] The role of CYP2D6 in the metabolism of amitriptyline is particularly significant given common polymorphisms for the 2D6 isozyme, which cause slow metabolism. In the future, genetic testing for these polymorphisms may help anticipate these issues and guide rational pharmacology.[33] Codeine is also strongly affected by the CYP2D6 isozyme, and when the patient either has the poor metabolizer phenotype or is functionally a poor metabolizer ("phenocopy") due to the presence of a 2D6 inhibitor, he or she will have difficulty metabolizing codeine to its morphine metabolite and therefore not get adequate pain relief.[34] These interactions must be taken into account to minimize the risk of respiratory arrest due to overdosing/undermetabolizing an opioid analgesic.

An additional mechanism by which pain medicines can interact with tricyclic antidepressants is the risk of QT interval prolongation, potentially resulting in torsades de pointes. Although methadone is the opioid most known clinically for causing this problem, other opioids such as oxycodone and buprenorphine have been shown to prolong the QT interval somewhat.[35] When combined with psychiatric medications such as tricyclic antidepressants, which are well known to cause QT interval prolongation due to their effect on ion channels, there is an increased risk of synergism causing a dangerously long QT interval and increased risk of torsades de pointes.[36]

Patients already treated with chronic methadone or buprenorphine may continue this treatment if hospitalized. However, increased doses of methadone to relieve pain may result in excessively high doses with risk of side effects such as sedation and nausea, as well as prolongation of the QT interval. In addition, methadone maintenance treatment is given once a day in the methadone clinic, while methadone treatment of pain is generally given multiple times a day.[37]

Buprenorphine maintenance is a safe and effective outpatient treatment for opioid addiction; however, it is less helpful in pain management, especially in acute pain management, because it has both high receptor binding affinity for the mu-opioid receptor and a pronounced "ceiling effect" due to its partial agonist status, limiting the amount of analgesic effect available.[38] Alford et al.[39] described three approaches to this problem: increasing the dosage and the frequency of dosing up to three times a day, but not more than 32 mg/day; adding a short-acting full agonist to improve pain relief; and finally, converting the patient from buprenorphine to a full agonist long-acting opioid for a period of time. Buprenorphine can also be administered in a transdermal form for chronic pain and has been used both acute and long term use in Europe with good results.[40]

Neuropathy Management

With the widespread use of HAART, peripheral neuropathies have become the most common neurologic complication of HIV infection.[41] Distal symmetric polyneuropathy (DSPN) accounts for 90% of all HIV neuropathy, which in turn constitutes 5% to 20% of all neurologic complications of HIV infection.[42] Although the neuropathy is often symmetric, it may be predominately on one side or involve one or more of the spinal nerve roots. Patients may experience spontaneous pain and paresthesias, at times severe. It is advisable to test for the presence of HIV-1 antibodies in all patients with acquired demyelinating neuropathies who have conceivable HIV-1 risk factors or suspicious laboratory test results, such as cerebrospinal fluid pleocytosis, positive hepatitis B titers, or polyclonal gammaglobulinemia.[43]

Neuropathic pain is generally better treated with adjuvant medications such as nortriptyline, gabapentin, pregabalin, or carbamazepine; however, initial pain treatment with short-acting analgesics may provide some immediate relief before the adjuvant medications take effect. Opioid analgesics should be reserved for patients with severe pain and low abuse risk. A review of 174 studies of neuropathic pain showed that tricyclic antidepressants, serotonin-noradrenaline reuptake inhibitors (SNRIs), the anticonvulsants gabapentin and pregabalin, and opioids are the drug classes for which there is the best evidence for a clinically relevant effect.[44] In one small study,[45] patients on methadone (and coanalgesics) for 12 months to treat chronic neuropathic pain noted an average of 43% pain relief (range 0% to 80%), 47% improvement in quality of life (range 0% to 100%), and 30% improvement in sleep (range 0% to 60%). Methadone was effective at relieving pain and ameliorating quality of life and sleep in 62% of patients.

Ethical Issues

It is the pain doctor's goal to improve "life that is not worth living." Ethics refers to moral principles embraced by an individual or group designed to provide rules for *right* conduct.[46] According to James Giordano, ethicist for the American Society of Interventional Pain Physicians (ASIPP), the ethical crisis in pain care necessitates a three-step process: identification of the problems, critical evaluation of various ethical systems, and "a description of how the structure and function of the practice—as a social good—might be enacted within a paradigm of (somewhat) non-hegemonious, integrative pain care."[47]

The prescribing of opioids is fraught with dangers for physician and patient alike. For patients, the risk of inappropriate use of opioids includes the risks of adverse side effects, ineffective (or less than optimally effective) pain management, problems of opioid tolerance and refractoriness, and in some cases even opioid addiction.[48] However, in a 2007 review, Ballantyne called upon pain providers to better understand that opioid therapy has relatively small risks of prosecution and addiction and, as such, must be more accurately considered against the effects that chronic uncontrolled pain has on an individual.[49] At the most fundamental level, improving pain management is simply the right thing to do. As a tangible expression of compassion, it is a cornerstone of health care's humanitarian mission.

Review of the anesthesia closed claim system showed that medication management issues represented 17% of 295 chronic noncancer pain claims.[50] Most patients were prescribed opioids (94%) and also additional psychoactive medications (58%). Eighty percent of patients had at least one factor commonly associated with medication misuse, and 24% had multiple risk factors. Most claims (82%) involved either patients who did not cooperate in their care (69%) or inappropriate medication management by physicians (59%). Death was the most common outcome in medication management claims. Alleged addiction from prescribed opioids was the complaint in 24%.

Koeppe et al.[2] noted that lower socioeconomic status (as measured by lack of private health insurance), injection drug use (IDU) as a risk factor for HIV, and a history of prior physical or emotional abuse had a high association with opioid use for pain relief. They felt that these observations were consistent with data from the HIV-negative population showing relationships between psychosocial issues, pain, and opioid use.[51] Their conclusion was that, although HIV and its medications may be involved in the etiology of chronic pain, psychosocial variables that are highly concentrated in the HIV-positive population might also be responsible for a significant amount of the pain and opioid use. This implies a use of opioids not for pain relief per se but for self-medication of anxiety and depression.

In clinical practice, a significant proportion of the patients suffering with inadequate pain control also have risk factors, such as past substance abuse or psychiatric comorbidity. As in many cases in medical ethics, there are mixed situations where the mandate to help and the mandate to "do no harm" can potentially come into conflict. Untreated, unmanageable pain is clearly a grave harm to the patient. At the same time, iatrogenic opioid addiction is a harmful state and the physician must take appropriate care when treating a patient who is at increased risk for developing this complication. With the recent increase in both opioid abuse and opioid diversion, greater concern is being expressed by society at large, and physicians may feel concern that they are risking censure or legal penalty by prescribing opioids. Denying patients opioids may also have foreseeable adverse consequences, including untreated pain, disability, and increased risk of doctor shopping, seeking more care in emergency departments, or obtaining opioids illegally.

It is incumbent on the physician to determine the balance of risk and benefit for each individual patient before making treatment decisions.[52] It is also necessary to reduce the risk as much as possible by using best practices, limiting dosage and duration, and determining the patient's risk factors prior to treatment. Complex cases may require referral to a pain specialist; however, providers may also be able to manage many more challenging patients with some education and consistent access to supervision by a specialist pain physician. Project ECHO, which uses telemedicine to help academic specialists comanage complex patients in rural settings with their primary care providers, is a model for this and is now being used to provide patients in Washington, Illinois, and New Mexico with specialty care in the fields of hepatitis C infection,[53] chronic pain, and other complex medical issues.

Initial Recommendations

Although Mr. N has been on gabapentin in the past, a significant number of patients have not had adequate trials of anticonvulsants such as gabapentin. In one author's experience (AMT, personal communication), more than 50% of patients seen in her clinic who have "failed" gabapentin were never on doses higher than 900 mg. Clinical randomized trials have confirmed that doses of 1,800 to 3,600 mg/day are necessary for neuropathic pain treatment.[54] Therefore, the patient needs to be interviewed further to determine the maximum dose of gabapentin previously tried and any side effects that limited its dose escalation.

Given Mr. N's history of substance abuse, close monitoring will be imperative when proposing opioid management. A LAO would be most appropriate, and methadone, with its long half-life, NMDA inhibition, and use in SUD seems the most appropriate choice of opioid. No particular set amount of methadone can be recommended, because ART treatment may involve the use of medications that are CYP3A4 and CYP2D6 inhibitors (which will increase methadone levels) as well as inducers (which will potentially decrease levels).

These interactions may directly affect the dosing of antiretroviral medications, so it is essential to develop a collaborative relationship between the pain provider and the primary care provider for the patient with HIV. A recent study has shown a limited knowledge base about opioid prescribing and opioid misuse among HIV treatment providers, so this relationship may be conceived as an interaction between two providers with only limited knowledge of each other's fields.[55] It is not uncommon for patients to change HAART regimens for a variety of reasons, so early discussion with the HIV treatment provider may allow the treatment to sidestep potential interactions through a change of HIV medications.

Psychological evaluation and subsequent appropriate treatment of potential depression and anxiety will also be important issues to address. However, many antidepressants (such as fluoxetine, paroxetine, bupropion, and duloxetine)[56,57] are CYP2D6 inhibitors, and again the potential for altered opioid blood levels exists.

Long-Term Plan

The methadone should be titrated slowly (perhaps as little as a 10-mg/day increase per month) until pain relief or intolerable side effects occur. In a longitudinal study of 106 HIV patients, methadone patients on ART reported fewer side effects than buprenorphine patients on ART.[58] The most common side effects of opioids[59] are usually manageable:

- Nausea usually clears over time spontaneously but may be managed with antinausea medications such as metoclopramide and promethazine
- Constipation occurs in 40% to 95% of patients treated with opioids and, unlike other side effects, does not improve over time.[60] Bulk laxatives, bowel stimulants, and oral opioid antagonists can be useful.
- Switching opioids and/or routes of administration may provide benefits for patients.

Because methadone blood levels can change drastically with changes in medications, very close collaboration between the pain physician and the infectious disease physician will be necessary to avoid disastrous (and potentially lethal) swings in methadone blood levels that can occur with changes in metabolism of methadone.

Summary Points

HIV patients are highly likely to develop pain, both from HIV infection directly and from associated factors. They may not get adequate pain treatment, yet pain control is a factor in their survival. Opioid treatment, while more problematic than had been previously hoped, is still essential to pain management. Patients who appear likely to benefit from opioid therapy, or who have previously responded well to this therapy, should not be excluded from consideration without careful assessment and, in some cases, consultation with a pain specialist. Pain management needs to be highly individualized in these patients. In particular, it is important to identify specific pain syndromes that may respond better to nonopioid treatment, such as injection therapy. When the decision has been made to start or continue opioid treatment, it is necessary to gather a complete history, especially the medication history and any psychiatric and substance history. It is advisable to develop clear communication between the pain management prescriber and the provider treating the HIV and related conditions, as HIV regimens are both complex and subject to change. It is clear that patients with past substance abuse histories are much more likely to develop aberrant pain treatment behaviors than those without, but with proper precautions, even challenging patients can be treated with a high degree of safety and security. Finally, it is important to note that opioid replacement therapy is very helpful for many opioid-addicted patients with HIV and must be taken into account when developing a plan of care for their pain conditions.

References

1. Larue F, Fontaine A, Colleau SM. Underestimation and undertreatment of pain in HIV disease: multicentre study. *BMJ*. 1997;314(7073):23–28.

2. Koeppe J, Armon C, Lyda K, Nielsen C, Johnson S. . Ongoing pain despite aggressive opioid pain management among persons with HIV. *Clin J Pain*. 2010;26(3):190–198.

3. Tsao J, Stein J, Dobalian A. Pain, problem drug use history, and aberrant analgesic use behaviors in persons living with HIV. *Pain*. 2007;133(1–3):128–137.

4. Tsao J, Dobalian A, Stein J. Illness burden mediates the relationship between pain and illicit drug use in persons living with HIV. *Pain*. 2005;119(1–3):124–132.

5. Jan SA. Introduction: landscape of opioid dependence. *J Manag Care Pharm*. 2010;16(1 Suppl B):S4–S8.

6. Fleming MF, Davis J, Passik SD. Reported lifetime aberrant drug-taking behaviors are predictive of current substance use and mental health problems in primary care patients. *Pain Med*. 2008;9(8):1098–1106.

7. Ives TJ, Chelminski PR, Hammett-Stabler CA, et al. Predictors of opioid misuse in patients with chronic pain: a prospective cohort study. *BMC Health Serv Res*. 2006;6:46.

8. Nicholson B, Passik SD. Management of chronic noncancer pain in the primary care setting. *South Med J.* 2007;100(10):1028–1036.

9. Trescot AM, Helm S, Hansen H, et al. Opioids in the management of chronic non-cancer pain: an update of American Society of the Interventional Pain Physicians' (ASIPP) Guidelines. *Pain Physician.* 2008;11(2 Suppl):S5–S62.

10. Von Korff, M., Merrill JO, Rutter CM, Sullivan M, Campbell CI, Weisner C. Time-scheduled vs. pain-contingent opioid dosing in chronic opioid therapy. *Pain.* 2011;152(6):1256–1262.

11. Walker JM, Farney RJ, Rhondeau SM, et al. Chronic opioid use is a risk factor for the development of central sleep apnea and ataxic breathing. *J Clin Sleep Med.* 2007;3(5):455–461.

12. Wynn G, Cozza K, Zapor M, Wortmann G, Armstrong S. Med-psych drug-drug interactions update. Antiretrovirals, part III: antiretrovirals and drugs of abuse. *Psychosomatics.* 2005;46(1):79–87.

13. Clay PG, Dong BJ, Sorensen SJ, Tseng A, Romanelli F, Antoniou T. Advances in human immunodeficiency virus therapeutics. *Ann Pharmacother.* 2006;40(4):704–709.

14. Trescot AM, Datta S, Lee M, Hansen H. Opioid pharmacology. *Pain Physician.* 2008;11(2 Suppl):S133–S153.

15. Gabrail NY, Dvergsten C, Ahdieh H. Establishing the dosage equivalency of oxymorphone extended release and oxycodone controlled release in patients with cancer pain: a randomized controlled study. *Curr Med Res Opin.* 2004;20(6):911–918.

16. Grond S, Sablotzki A. Clinical pharmacology of tramadol. *Clin Pharmacokinet.* 2004;43(13):879–923.

17. Gruber V, McCance-Katz E. Methadone, buprenorphine, and street drug interactions with antiretroviral medications. *Curr HIV/AIDS Rep.* 2010;7(3):152–160.

18. Kakuda TN, Scholler-Gyure M, Hoetelmans RM. Pharmacokinetic interactions between etravirine and non-antiretroviral drugs. *Clin Pharmacokinet.* 2011;50(1):25–39.

19. Kharasch E, Walker A, Whittington D, Hoffer C, Bedynek P. Methadone metabolism and clearance are induced by nelfinavir despite inhibition of cytochrome P4503A (CYP3A) activity. *Drug Alcohol Depend.* 2009;101(3):158–168.

20. Luthi B, Huttner A, Speck RF, Mueller NJ. Methadone-induced torsade de pointes after stopping lopinavir-ritonavir. *Eur J Clin Microbiol Infect Dis.* 2007;26(5):367–369.

21. Rainey P, Friedland G, McCance-Katz E, et al. Interaction of methadone with didanosine and stavudine. *J Acquir Immune Defic Syndr.* 2000;24(3):241–248.

22. McCance-Katz E, Rainey P, Jatlow P, Friedland G. Methadone effects on zidovudine disposition (AIDS Clinical Trials Group 262). *J Acquir Immune Defic Syndr Hum Retrovirol.* 1998;18(5):435–443.

23. Cruciani RA. Methadone: to ECG or not to ECG…That is still the question. *J Pain Symptom Manage.* 2008;36(5):545–552.

24. Chugh SS, Socoteanu C, Reinier K, Waltz J, Jui J, Gunson K. A community-based evaluation of sudden death associated with therapeutic levels of methadone. *Am J Med.* 2008;121(1):66–71.

25. McCance-Katz EF, Moody DE, Morse GD, et al. Interaction between buprenorphine and atazanavir or atazanavir/ritonavir. *Drug Alcohol Depend.* 2007;91(2–3):269–278.

26. Basu S, Bruce R, Barry D, Altice F. Pharmacological pain control for human immunodeficiency virus-infected adults with a history of drug dependence. *J Subst Abuse Treat.* 2007;32(4):399–409.

27. Hughes J, Bickel W, Higgins S. Buprenorphine for pain relief in a patient with drug abuse. *Am J Drug Alcohol Abuse.* 1991;17(4):451–455.

28. Umbricht A, Hoover D, Tucker M, Leslie J, Chaisson R, Preston K. Opioid detoxification with buprenorphine, clonidine, or methadone in hospitalized heroin-dependent patients with HIV infection. *Drug Alcohol Depend.* 2003;69(3):263–272.

29. Eap CB, Buclin T, Baumann P. Interindividual variability of the clinical pharmacokinetics of methadone: implications for the treatment of opioid dependence. *Clin Pharmacokinet.* 2002;41(14):1153–1193.

30. Davoli M, Bargagli AM, Perucci CA, et al. Risk of fatal overdose during and after specialist drug treatment: the VEdeTTE study, a national multi-site prospective cohort study. *Addiction.* 2007;102(12):1954–1959.

31. Wahlstrom A, Lenhammar L, Ask B, Rane A. Tricyclic antidepressants inhibit opioid receptor binding in human brain and hepatic morphine glucuronidation. *Pharmacol Toxicol.* 1994;75(1):23–27.

32. Bomsien S, Skopp G. An in vitro approach to potential methadone metabolic-inhibition interactions. *Eur J Clin Pharmacol.* 2007;63(9):821–827.

33. Steimer W, Zopf K, von Amelunxen S, et al. Amitriptyline or not, that is the question: pharmacogenetic testing of CYP2D6 and CYP2C19 identifies patients with low or high risk for side effects in amitriptyline therapy. *Clin Chem.* 2005;51(2):376–385.

34. Caraco Y, Sheller J, Wood AJ. Pharmacogenetic determination of the effects of codeine and prediction of drug interactions. *J Pharmacol Exp Ther.* 1996;278(3):1165–1174.

35. Fanoe S, Jensen GB, Sjogren P, Korsgaard MP, Grunnet M. Oxycodone is associated with dose-dependent QTc prolongation in patients and low-affinity inhibiting of hERG activity in vitro. *Br J Clin Pharmacol.* 2009;67(2):172–179.

36. Vieweg WV, Wood MA. Tricyclic antidepressants, QT interval prolongation, and torsade de pointes. *Psychosomatics.* 2004;45(5):371–377.

37. Ballantyne J, Mao J. Opioid therapy for chronic pain. *N Engl J Med.* 2003;349(20):1943–1953.

38. Basu S, et al. Models for integrating buprenorphine therapy into the primary HIV care setting. *Clin Infect Dis.* 2006;42(5):716–721.

39. Alford D, Compton P, Samet J. Acute pain management for patients receiving maintenance methadone or buprenorphine therapy. *Ann Intern Med.* 2006;144(2):127–134.

40. Likar R, Kayser H, Sittl R. Long-term management of chronic pain with transdermal buprenorphine: a multicenter, open-label, follow-up study in patients from three short-term clinical trials. *Clin Ther.* 2006;28(6):943–952.

41. Nicholas PK, Kemppainen JK, Canaval GE, et al. Symptom management and self-care for peripheral neuropathy in HIV/AIDS. *AIDS Care.* 2007;19(2):179–189.

42. Willoughby R. Cerebellar ataxia, transverse myelitis and myopathy, Guillain-Barré, neuritis, and neuropathy. In: L. SS, ed. *Principles and practice of pediatric infectious diseases*. Philadelphia: Churchill Livingstone; 2009:322–325.

43. Harati Y, Bosch E. Disorders of peripheral nerves. In: Bradley W, et al., eds. *Neurology in clinical practice*. Philadelphia: Butterwork-Heinemann; 2008:2249–2345.

44. Finnerup NB, Otto M, McQuay HJ, Jensen TS, Sindrup SH. Algorithm for neuropathic pain treatment: an evidence based proposal. *Pain*. 2005;118(3):289–305.

45. Altier N, Dion D, Boulanger A, Choiniere M. Management of chronic neuropathic pain with methadone: a review of 13 cases. *Clin J Pain*. 2005;21(4):364–369.

46. Novy DM, Ritter LM, McNeill J. A primer of ethical issues involving opioid therapy for chronic nonmalignant pain in a multidisciplinary setting. *Pain Med*. 2009;10(2):356–363.

47. Giordano J. Ethics of, and in, pain medicine: constructs, content, and contexts of application. *Pain Physician*. 2008;11(4):391–392.

48. Trescot AM. Ethical considerations in interventional pain management. In: Van Norman G, ed. *Clinical ethics in anesthesiology*. New York: Cambridge University Press; 2011:137–142.

49. Ballantyne JC. Opioid analgesia: perspectives on right use and utility. *Pain Physician*. 2007;10(3):479–491.

50. Fitzgibbon DR Rathmell JP, Michna E, Stephens LS, Posner KL, Domino KB. Malpractice claims associated with medication management for chronic pain. *Anesthesiology*. 2010;112(4):948–956.

51. Sullivan MD, Edlund MJ, Zhang L, Unutzer J, Wells KB. Association between mental health disorders, problem drug use, and regular prescription opioid use. *Arch Intern Med*. 2006;166(19):2087–2093.

52. Giordano J. Changing the practice of pain medicine writ large and small through identifying problems and establishing goals. *Pain Physician*. 2006;9(4):283–285.

53. Arora S, et al. Academic health center management of chronic diseases through knowledge networks: Project ECHO. *Acad Med*. 2007;82(2):154–160.

54. Backonja M, Glanzman RL. Gabapentin dosing for neuropathic pain: evidence from randomized, placebo-controlled clinical trials. *Clin Ther*. 2003;25(1):81–104.

55. Lum PJ, Little S, Botsko M, et al. Opioid-prescribing practices and provider confidence recognizing opioid analgesic abuse in HIV primary care settings. *J Acquir Immune Defic Syndr*. 2011;56(Suppl 1):S91–S97.

56. Preskorn SH, Greenblatt DJ, Flockhart D, et al. Comparison of duloxetine, escitalopram, and sertraline effects on cytochrome P450 2D6 function in healthy volunteers. *J Clin Psychopharmacol*. 2007;27(1):28–34.

57. Kotlyar M, Brauer LH, Tracy TS, et al. Inhibition of CYP2D6 activity by bupropion. *J Clin Psychopharmacol*. 2005;25(3):226–229.

58. Carrieri MP, Roux P, Cohen J, et al. Self-reported side effects in buprenorphine and methadone patients receiving antiretroviral therapy: results from the MANIF 2000 cohort study. *Addiction*. 2010;105(12):2160–2168.

59. Benyamin R, Trescot AM, Datta S, et al. Opioid complications and side effects. *Pain Physician*. 2008;11(2 Suppl):S105–S120.

60. Swegle JM, Logemann C. Management of common opioid-induced adverse effects. *Am Fam Physician*. 2006;74(8):1347–1354.

Chapter 10

United States Workers' Compensation and Disability

James P. Robinson

The Case

Bob Benson is a 42-year-old man who has done deliveries for FedEx for the past 15 years. He has no history of work injuries. On the day of injury, he reports abrupt onset of low back pain (LBP) with radiation into the right lower extremity (RLE) while lifting a heavy box. Two days later he sees his primary care provider (PCP), who has cared for him for the past 8 years. The PCP files a workers' compensation claim for Bob and agrees to function as attending physician for the claim. Bob is prescribed diclofenac 75 mg twice daily and hydrocodone (5 mg/500 acetaminophen) three times daily as needed for pain. He is seen on a weekly basis over the next 4 weeks and continues to report disabling pain. His hydrocodone/acetaminophen dose is increased, reaching four tablets at double the opioid dose (10 mg/325 acetaminophen) per day by 1 month after injury. His PCP refers him to an orthopedist, who recommends decompressive surgery at L5-S1, and has Bob undergo evaluation by a pain specialist colleague. The pain specialist concludes that Bob is undermedicated and switches him to a combination of OxyContin 20 mg bid plus oxycodone 5 mg 4 times daily for breakthrough pain. Bob undergoes surgery 3 months after injury. This leads to some improvement in his RLE pain, but he continues to report severe disabling LBP postoperatively. The orthopedist says nothing more can be done surgically. The pain specialist continues Bob on the aforementioned OxyContin/oxycodone regimen for 3 months postoperatively but then says he must turn over management to the PCP. The PCP takes over Bob's opioid prescribing. Six months after surgery, Bob is sent to an independent medical examination (IME) by the workers' compensation (WC) claim manager. The examiners judge him to be employable, so his time loss payments are discontinued. Also, they report that they can find no evidence that the patient's OxyContin/oxycodone regimen has improved his functional status and so the WC carrier then informs the PCP that it will no longer pay for any opioid therapy. Because of the financial burden of the costly OxyContin (typically greater than $100 per month), the PCP switches the patient to the much cheaper methadone 5 mg 3 times daily (typically less than $20 per month). After the IME, the patient indicates that he might be able to do the job he had at the time of injury, but only if he has ongoing access to opioids. Because he has already been terminated by his employer, FedEx, at the time of injury, Bob seeks employment in package delivery with three other companies. All three tell him that they maintain drug-free workplaces and will insist on urine drug testing as a condition of employment. He then tells them that he has a prescription for methadone to treat pain. None of the companies offers him a job. The patient suspects that he is rejected because he is using methadone, although none of the prospective employers actually states this. After 6 months of seeking employment, the patient finally is hired for an entry-level position as a receptionist for a law firm.

List of Considerations

- Coordination between PMD and pain specialist regarding opioid therapy
- Regulations and expectations that result from a patient's participation in a typical US workers' compensation system
- Barriers to return to work for people on opioids

Clinical Discussion

When opioids are used in acute care settings, it does not matter whether the patient has a work injury or some other kind of medical problem. Thus, the patient with a tibial fracture from a skiing accident will be treated the same as the one with a tibial fracture from a fall at work. But if physicians contemplate providing long-term opioid therapy for patients, they need to consider differences between WC patients and ones with other kinds of health insurance. The discussion to follow is relevant only to long-term use of opioids in WC patients.

Physicians typically think of pain and appropriate pain treatment as clinical issues. But pain treatment always occurs in a social context. One key element of this context is the insurance system that pays for a patient's treatment.

As all clinicians know, there is a plethora of health insurance carriers and insurance programs in the United States. For purposes of the present discussion, they will be bundled into two large groups. One group consists of health insurance provided by US private insurance companies (such as Aetna) and the two major US government insurance programs—Medicaid and Medicare. In the discussion to follow, these will be called general health insurance programs (GHIPs). WC makes up the other group. This typology leaves out some circumstances (e.g., the arrangements for coverage provided following motor vehicle accidents) and glosses over substantial differences among programs in the two groups. But it highlights special features of WC programs.

GHIPs pay the professional fees of health care providers and also pay for various ancillary charges related to medical care, such as laboratory tests. When contrasted with WC programs, they have three key common features. First, GHIPs cover costs for essentially all of a patient's medical problems (unless there are exclusions for some, such as riders for preexisting conditions). Second, they do not provide wage replacement for patients whose medical problems prevent them from working. Essentially, a patient's work status makes no difference, unless a patient with insurance benefits through work becomes unable to work, and thus suffers loss of the private health insurance plan. In this event, the insurance carrier does not incur any financial liability—it simply stops paying for the patient's care. Third, GHIPs typically provide open-ended benefits. As long as a beneficiary remains employed and pays his or her share of the premiums, he or she can receive care indefinitely.

In the United States, WC systems exist in each of the 50 states. In addition, there are two federal workers' compensation systems, and a separate program for Washington D.C.[1,2] There are significant differences among these programs, but there are also several key features that are common to all of them and distinguish them from GHIPs.

1. WC provides benefits only for work-related conditions. Thus, when a worker reports symptoms, a judgment must be made not only about the nature of the underlying medical problem but also about whether or not the problem arose "out of and in the course of employment"[2] (see p. 10).

2. Compensation systems assume responsibility not only for the medical care of an injured worker but also for his or her ability to work. Thus, WC carriers provide time loss payments for workers who are temporarily incapacitated because of injury and often vocational services once the workers have reached maximal medical improvement. They also provide pensions for those workers who continue to be incapacitated after maximal improvement has been achieved. An important consequence of this mandate is that treating physicians are repeatedly required to evaluate the work capabilities of injured workers (IWs), and WC systems may refuse to pay for symptomatic treatment that does not demonstrably promote the IWs' return to work.

3. WC programs are conceptualized as temporary insurance programs. They operate under the assumption that recovery after injury follows a fairly predictable course, such that an IW initially shows progressive improvement and then reaches a plateau. In compensation law, a worker is said to be "fixed and stable" or to have reached "maximal medical improvement" when he or she plateaus. At this juncture, US compensation law generally dictates that medical treatment be terminated and that a decision regarding the worker's employability be made. Also, the worker is entitled to a cash settlement based on his or her permanent partial impairment when he or she reaches maximal medical improvement.

In part because of their different mandates, WC carriers require much more documentation from treating physicians than GHIPs. Treating physicians need to be prepared for challenges to their treatment plans and pressure to focus their treatment on the goal of return to work as quickly as possible.[3] This pressure is apparent in relation to Bob's opioid therapy.

As described in other chapters of this book, the goals of opioid therapy can often be classified into two broad groups. When the goal is pain palliation, a patient's report that he or she is experiencing significant relief from opioid therapy may be sufficient to justify continued treatment, irrespective of functional recovery. When the goal is functional recovery, the physician needs to be attentive to improvement in the patient's ability to carry out tasks. WC carriers pressure physicians to focus on the second goal. As seen in the Bob's history, WC carriers sometimes refuse to pay for treatments that do not demonstrably contribute to improvement in a patient's functional capabilities.

A physician who contemplates long-term opioid therapy for an IW should be aware that the efficacy of such therapy in the context of work injuries is questionable. While randomized controlled trials provide reasonably persuasive evidence that opioids taken over a period of a few weeks reduce pain, evidence from these trials for functional improvement (including return to work) from opioid therapy is much less impressive. These issues are discussed in other chapters of the present volume (chapters 2, 5 and 9) and will not be discussed here. But the sobering evidence from randomized controlled trials implies that physicians should be aware of the possibility that opioids will not necessarily help IWs return to their jobs.

Evidence from WC carriers also should give the clinician pause about the efficacy of opioids for IWs. Four recent studies have shown that IWs who receive opioids are likely to remain disabled for longer time periods than ones who do not receive opioids.[4–7] Thus, in these studies, opioid therapy could be viewed as a risk factor for prolonged disability. It should be noted that research based on large WC databases can be misleading. In the present instance, one could argue that IWs with more severe problems are relatively likely to receive opioids, and that severity of injury is the driving force behind both use of opioids and delayed recovery. For example, Gross et al.[5] state: "As expected, claimants with more severe injuries were more likely to receive opioids. An association was observed between early opioid prescription and delayed recovery, however, this is likely explained by pain severity or other unmeasured confounders" (p. 525). Thus, while the findings from WC database studies are not conclusive, they certainly challenge the effectiveness of opioids in facilitating functional recovery in IWs.

As Bob's case demonstrates, another problem associated with long-term opioid therapy in IWs is that the WC carrier might construe the treatment as palliative, and therefore refuse to continue paying for the medications.

Finally, even if an IW on opioid therapy reports pain relief, improves functionally, and appears to be ready to return to work, continued opioid therapy may act as a barrier to his or her successful return to work. Issues related to the ability of IWs on opioids to return to work divide into two groups: impairment in work activities secondary to opioid use and unwillingness of employers to hire IWs on opioids.

Opioids, Impairment, and Ability to Work

A considerable amount of research effort has been devoted to the possibility that opioids cause impairments that interfere with work. For simplicity, these efforts can be divided into two groups: research on "component" skills/behaviors needed to engage in virtually any kind of work (alertness, cognitive function, motor function) and research on functional activities that are integral to at least some kinds of work. Because of the enormous heterogeneity of work activities, only a tiny proportion of these functional activities have been studied among opioid users. The discussion to follow focuses on two such activities—safety in walking (absence of falls) and safety in driving.

With regard to component skills/behaviors, it is reasonable to assume that most jobs require alertness, normal cognitive functioning, and normal ability to perform skilled motor tasks. Each of these component processes has been studied in relation to opioid use.

Sedation is felt to be a common side effect of opioid use and has been shown to be problematic in selected populations of patients with pain—including cancer patients, elderly patients, patients with various medical comorbidities, and hospitalized patients.[8–11] But among patients without comorbidities, it is widely believed that while sedation frequently occurs at the onset of opioid therapy and in response to dose escalations, it is not a major problem for patients on stable regimens. McNicol et al.[12] state the issue as follows: "Sedation most frequently occurs at initiation of opioid therapy or when a significant dose increase occurs. Sedation is associated with transient drowsiness or cognitive impairment. Symptoms frequently resolve after a few days" (p. 233).

Cognitive functioning among opioid users has been assessed via a wide range of tests, such as the Digit Span, Trail Making, Digit Symbol, and Hopkins Verbal Learning tests. It is logical to assume that cognitive impairment should be common among opioid users, because sedation interferes with cognitive functions. However, research on the existence and severity of cognitive impairment associated with opioids has been inconclusive.[13] In fact, there is some evidence that cognitive functioning improves on opioids, perhaps because of the pain reduction that the medications provide.[14]

Research on motor function among opioid users has relied on vigilance tasks, reaction time tasks, and tracking tasks, among others.[15,16] As with cognitive functioning, it is logical to assume that opioids might cause impairment secondary to their sedative effects. This has in fact been found in animal studies.[17] However, research on the effects of opioids on motor functioning among humans has produced inconsistent results.[15,16]

As far as functional activities are concerned, one area that has been examined is safety in ambulation, as manifested by absence of falls. Research has revealed that among elderly people, ones taking opioids are at increased risk for falls.[18,19] Driving safety is another domain that has been studied in detail. Research to date is inconclusive. There is no convincing evidence that in the aggregate patients on stable doses of opioids are unsafe as drivers.[20] However, some patients are likely to be impaired. Chou[21] summarizes the situation as follows:

> In the absence of signs or symptoms of impairment, there is no evidence that patients maintained on stable doses of COT [chronic opioid therapy] should be restricted from driving .... Nonetheless, opioids may cause somnolence, clouded mentation, decreased concentration, and slower reflexes or incoordination. Clinicians should counsel all patients initially prescribed COT not to drive or engage in potentially dangerous work or other activities when impaired. Patients should be educated about the greater risk of impairment when starting opioid therapy, when increasing doses, and when taking other drugs or substances that may have central nervous effects, including alcohol. (p. 474)

The research summarized here falls far short of providing definitive answers to questions about the impairing effects of opioids or about the implications of these effects for the ability of IWs to return to work. Any attempt to provide definitive answers runs into a host of methodologic and conceptual problems. A short list includes the following: (a) Patients are more likely to be impaired during initiation of opioid therapy than after they have had a chance to adapt to their opioids. This issue limits the validity of comparisons between patients on chronic opioid therapy and normal volunteers who are opioid naïve. (b) Severe pain can limit a person's ability to perform work-related activities. Thus, assuming that an opioid is helpful in reducing a patient's pain, the question is whether the adverse effects of the opioid offset the benefit of more effective pain relief. (c) "Cognitive functioning" refers to an extraordinarily broad set of behaviors and capabilities, as does "motor functioning." Given the diversity of specific behaviors/skills underlying these broad rubrics, one should anticipate inconsistencies among studies purporting to study them. (d) Research on the effects of opioids on work-related functions typically takes place over short periods of time. Patients on opioids may be able to rally and perform well during these short testing sessions. But actual work requires diligence and persistence over extended periods of time. It is quite possible that workers on opioids have difficulty sustaining high levels of performance, even if they are able to perform well for short periods of time. (e) There is enormous variation in the jobs that workers carry out. Common sense suggests that opioids are likely to be more problematic for some types of work than for others.

In the absence of definitive evidence about what job-related tasks patients on opioids can carry out, prudence dictates that physicians treating IWs with opioids be aware of the potential adverse effects of the medications on work activities and take steps to mitigate them. A key issue is that they need to be aware of the fact that patients differ with respect to impairment from opioids.

Consequently, some might be severely impaired, even if research does not support the presence of impairment in the majority of opioid users. As far as mitigation is concerned, physicians should avoid changing patients' opioid regimens while they are attempting to reintegrate into the workforce. Also, they need to assess the extent to which IWs perceive themselves as impaired because of their opioids. Third, they should warn patients that they can suffer significant consequences if they make errors at work because of impairment caused by opioid use.

Workplace Barriers for Injured Workers on Opioids

It is difficult to judge the frequency with which IWs are denied opportunities to return to work because of their opioids. Private industry and governments at the federal and state level in the United States have initiated multiple programs to create drug-free workplaces.[22] For example, the Drug Free Workplace Act of 1988 required organizations that contract with the federal government to establish programs to reduce drug abuse by employees.[23] As one component of programs to reduce inappropriate use of illicit drugs and alcohol, many companies have required employees to undergo urine drug tests.[24,25]

Discussions about drug-free workplaces are routinely framed in terms of the need to prevent workers from using illicit substances, psychoactive substances that have not been prescribed for them, or excessive alcohol. The status of prescription opioids is ambiguous. For example, in a recent publication entitled *What Employees Need to Know about DOT Drug and Alcohol Testing*, the US Department of Transportation (DOT)[26] stated: "Prescription medicine and OTC drugs may be allowed" (p. 3). This document then lists requirements that must be met for a patient on prescription medications to engage in safety-sensitive work for the DOT. One requirement is that the prescribing physician indicate that the medication "is consistent with the safe performance of your duties." But the DOT makes clear that meeting the stated requirements may not be sufficient, because subsidiary organizations within the DOT might establish different standards regarding opioids. As an example of this, the Federal Aviation Administration, a subsidiary of the DOT, does not permit pilots to use any prescription opioid.[27]

Given the myriad of policies employed by US governmental organizations and private companies, it is difficult to know how likely it is that a patient's job application will be compromised by his or her use of prescription opioids. To make matters more complicated, cases regarding the rights of opioid users in the workplace are currently being litigated.[28] The balance between an employer's right to maintain a safe, drug-free work environment and an employee's privacy rights and right to work while using medications sanctioned by his or her physician has not been determined in the US court system.

In theory, at least according to the US Equal Employment Opportunity Administration, applicants for jobs do not need to provide information about their prescription medications.[29] But the practicality of this protection of privacy is vitiated by the fact that employers have the right to demand urine drug testing before an applicant is accepted for a job.[29] Thus, prospective employers can learn that a job candidate is using opioids. Although urine drug testing is supposed to be deferred until after an applicant has been assured of a job, this safeguard can easily be circumvented. In the case given in this chapter, Bob quite reasonably responded to the demand for drug testing by telling prospective employers that he was using methadone.

No systematic research exists on the ways in which prospective employers respond to information that job applicants are taking prescription opioids. But evidence from the mental health arena suggests that prospective employers might reject such applicants. Research on individuals with mental impairments indicates that potential employers frequently refuse to make job offers after they learn about the impairments.[30] It is very likely that people meet the same prejudice when they indicate to a potential employer that they have chronic pain and that they take opioids for the pain.

In summary, although the implications of prescription opioids for reintegration into the workforce are not entirely clear, physicians need to be aware that when they treat IWs with long-term opioids, they may well be prejudicing the chances of the IWs to reenter the work force. In the case example, Bob had a poor vocational outcome. He was able to return to work, but in a position that offered him much less money than the job he had at the time of injury.

Ethical Issues

In one sense, the use of opioids in WC patients presents no ethical issues above and beyond those raised by prescribing the medications for other groups of patients. But, as with any intervention, a physician has an obligation to be knowledgeable about the harms and benefits of opioid therapy in the WC setting. As described previously, IWs on opioids face risks because of the actions of their WC carrier, and also because of the responses they might encounter by prospective employers when they attempt to return to work. Thus, the ethical mandate is for a physician treating an IW to be aware of these special risks and to take them into account when he or she decides whether to prescribe long-term opioids.

Initial Recommendations

The most appropriate course of action for Bob's PCP would be to refer him to a multidisciplinary pain rehabilitation program. Such a program would help in at least two ways. First, it would help the patient regain physical capabilities and deal with various psychological barriers to reactivation and reemployment. Second, the program would include a systematic opioid taper, with an important goal of having Bob completely off opioids by the end of the program, thereby increasing his employment opportunities.

Long-Term Plan

Assuming Bob successfully completed a pain rehabilitation program, had substantially improved physical capacities, and was off opioids, the role of the PCP would be to encourage and strongly support these improvements. This is often not a simple matter. Patients who appear to have benefited greatly from pain rehabilitation programs sometimes regress substantially over a period of months after they complete the programs. As one indication of this regression, they often make demands on PCPs to reinstate their opioid therapy. In this difficult situation, it is helpful for the PCP to maintain regular contact with the treatment team at the rehabilitation facility, so they can work together to reinforce the gains that the patient made while going through the rehabilitation program.

Summary Points

Opioid therapy for patients with workers' compensation claims presents challenges over and above those presented by opioid therapy for other patient groups. Physicians who prescribe opioids for IWs need to be aware of these.

One set of challenges stems from the rules and policies of WC carriers. These often differ from rules and policies of other insurers. For example, WC carriers may stop paying for treatments (including opioids) that do not promote return to work. Other challenges relate to the effects of opioid therapy upon return to work among IWs. A basic principle is that a treatment program for an injured worker must focus on interventions that facilitate his or her return to work. This is mandated by WC carriers, and also is in the best interest of the IW. If the treatment program includes long-term opioid therapy, the treating physician needs to understand the implications of such therapy for return to work. Research has addressed the effects of opioids on several work-related activities, including alertness, cognitive functioning, motor functioning, safety in walking, and safety in driving. Although this research has been largely inconclusive, physicians need to be aware that these and other work-related functions can be impaired by opioids. Physicians should also be aware that large-scale research using WC databases has consistently shown that opioid therapy is associated with prolongation of work disability.

Finally, IWs on long-term opioid therapy may face challenges returning to work even when their pain is under good control and they are functioning well. The reason for this is that prospective employers who want drug-free workplaces might refuse to hire them.

References

1. *1998 Analysis of workers' compensation laws.* Washington, DC: U.S. Chamber of Commerce; 1998.

2. Williams CA. *An international comparison of workers' compensation.* Boston: Kluwer Academic Publishers; 1991.

3. Parry T. *Medical benefit delivery—group medical versus workers' compensation in California.* San Francisco: California Workers' Compensation Institute; 1994.

4. Volinn E, Jamison DF, Fine PG. Opioid therapy for nonspecific low back pain and the outcome of chronic work loss. *Pain.* 2009;142(3):194–201.

5. Gross DP, Stephens B, Bhambhani Y, et al. Opioid prescriptions in Canadian workers' compensation claimants: prescription trends and associations between early prescription and future recovery. *Spine* 2009;34(5):525–531.

6. Franklin GM, Stover BD, Turner JA, et al. Early opioid prescription and subsequent disability among workers with back injuries: the Disability Risk Identification Study Cohort. *Spine* 2008;33(2):199–204.

7. Webster BS, Verma SK, Gatchel RJ. Relationship between early opioid prescribing for acute occupational low back pain and disability duration, medical costs, subsequent surgery and late opioid use. *Spine* 2007;32(19):2127–2132.

8. Plante GE, VanItallie TB. Opioids for cancer pain: the challenge of optimizing treatment. *Metabolism.* 2010;59(Suppl 1):S47–S52.

9. Kahan M, Wilson L, Mailis-Gagnon A, Srivastava A. Canadian guideline for safe and effective use of opioids for chronic noncancer pain: clinical summary for family physicians. Part 2: special populations. *Can Fam Physician.* 2011;57(11):1269–1276, e419–e428.

10. Smith H, Bruckenthal P. Implications of opioid analgesia for medically complicated patients. *Drugs Aging.* 2010;27(5):417–433.

11. Nisbet AT, Mooney-Cotter F. Comparison of selected sedation scales for reporting opioid-induced sedation assessment. *Pain Manag Nurs.* 2009;10(3):154–164.

12. McNicol E, Horowicz-Mehler N, Fisk RA, et al.; American Pain Society. Management of opioid side effects in cancer-related and chronic noncancer pain: a systematic review. *J Pain.* 2003;4(5):231–256.

13. Kendall SE, Sjøgren P, Pimenta CA, Højsted J, Kurita GP. The cognitive effects of opioids in chronic non-cancer pain. *Pain.* 2010;150(2):225–230.

14. Jamison RN, Schein JR, Vallow S, Ascher S, Vorsanger GJ, Katz NP. Neuropsychological effects of long-term opioid use in chronic pain patients. *J Pain Symptom Manage* 2003;26:913–921.

15. Allen GJ, Hartl TL, Duffany S, et al. Cognitive and motor function after administration of hydrocodone bitartrate plus ibuprofen, ibuprofen alone, or placebo in healthy subjects with exercise-induced muscle damage: a randomized, repeated-dose, placebo-controlled study. *Psychopharmacology (Berl).* 2003;166(3):228–233.

16. Dagtekin O, Gerbershagen HJ, Wagner W, et al. Assessing cognitive and psychomotor performance under long term treatment with transdermal buprenorphine in chronic non-cancer pain patients. *Anesth Analg.* 2007;105:1442–1448.

17. Craft RM. Sex differences in analgesic, reinforcing, discriminative, and motoric effects of opioids. *Exp Clin Psychopharmacol.* 2008;16(5):376–385.

18. Hass B, Lungershausen J, Hertel N, Poulsen Nautrup B, Kotowa W, Liedgens H. Cost-effectiveness of strong opioids focussing on the long-term effects of opioid-related fractures: a model approach. *Eur J Health Econ.* 2009;10(3):309–321.

19. Vestergaard P, Rejnmark L, Mosekilde L. Fracture risk associated with the use of morphine and opiates. *J Intern Med.* 2006;260(1):76–87.

20. Dassanayake T, Michie P, Carter G, Jones A. Effects of benzodiazepines, antidepressants and opioids on driving: a systematic review and meta-analysis of epidemiological and experimental evidence. *Drug Saf.* 2011;34(2):125–156.

21. Chou R. Clinical guidelines from the American Pain Society and the American Academy of Pain Medicine on the use of chronic opioid therapy in chronic noncancer pain: what are the key messages for clinical practice? *Pol Arch Med Wewn.* 2009;119(7–8):469–477.

22. www.drugfreeworkplace.org.

23. US Department of Labor. Drug-Free Workplace Act of 1988. http://www.dol.gov/elaws/asp/drugfree/screen4.htm (accessed February 19, 2012).

24. Bush DM. The U.S. mandatory guidelines for federal workplace drug testing programs: current status and future considerations. *Forensic Sci Int.* 2008;174:111–119.

25. Walsh JM. New technology and new initiatives in U.S. workplace testing. *Forensic Sci Int.* 2008;174:120–124.

26. *What employees need to know about DOT drug and alcohol testing.* Washington, DC: U.S. Department of Transportation, Office of the Secretary; 2005.

27. FAA accepted medications. http://www.leftseat.com/medcat1.htm

28. Drug testing poses quandary for employers. *New York Times,* October 24, 2010.

29. EEOC NOTICE Number 915.002 Date 10/10/95. http://www.eeoc.gov/policy/docs/preemp.html

30. Cook JA. Employment barriers for persons with psychiatric disabilities: Update of a report for the President's Commission. *Psychiatr Serv.* 2006;57:1391–1405.

Chapter 11

Using Measurement-Based Tools to Improve Pain Care

David J. Tauben

The Case

Alice Cluny is a 26-year-old woman with an 8-year history of pelvic pain, onset at age 18 years following the birth of her first child. She carried two further pregnancies, requiring intermittent hydrocodone for her persistent ill-defined pelvic and bladder symptoms. At age 23 years a laparoscopic diagnosis of endometriosis was made and she was treated with cauterization of suspect lesions without benefit. Follow-up laparoscopy showed no further pathology. Ongoing pelvic pain prompted several months of gynecologic surgeries: vestibulectomy, bilateral staged oophorectomy/salpingectomy, and finally hysterectomy. Pain persisted, and urologic diagnosis of interstitial cystitis was made, prompted by painful frequent culture-negative dysuria, a "suspicious" cystoscopic biopsy, and several courses of transurethral procedures and instillations followed by complications of urinary retention requiring urethral self-catheterization 4 times daily. During these urogynecologic treatments, she was treated with escalating doses of opioids: hydrocodone, then oxycodone, then morphine extended release, then OxyContin at a dose of 40 mg 3 times daily. She was also prescribed carisoprodol 350 mg 3 times daily and alprazolam 1 mg 3 times daily. Her primary care physician took over her opioid prescriptions after there was "nothing left for the specialists to do." The primary care physician became concerned about visits and calls requesting early refills and concurrent requests for pain medication by her other treating specialists, then discharged Alice from her practice for "addiction and drug-seeking behavior."

List of Considerations

- Complex chronic pain is a disorder that requires multisystem assessment.
- Difficult clinical challenges need ongoing measurement and tracking.
- Treatment selection and outcomes are improved with measurement-based care.

Clinical Discussion

This is a complex clinical situation that evolved from pelvic pain as a symptom of a gynecologic disease (endometriosis during pregnancy) into a nonspecific primary pain disorder that continued after multiple surgeries, prompting escalation of polypharmacy management including high-dose opioids combined with sedative/hypnotics. Additionally, this woman demonstrated significant aberrant behaviors that led to a diagnosis of addiction that disrupted her relationship with her primary care provider. Several crucial questions are raised:

- What is this patient's "pain diagnosis"?
- What other diagnostic tests would assist in diagnosis?
- How can a physician incorporate a more thorough pain assessment within the limited time allotted for an office-based primary care visit?
- How does longitudinal recording of pain measures direct and improve outcome?

Diagnosing and Managing a Complex Chronic Medical Disorder

Primary care physicians are trained to assess and manage complex diseases using multisystem assessment tools. For instance, diabetes mellitus is diagnosed not just with a history of polyuria/polydipsia, but by measuring fasting blood sugars, hemoglobin A_{1c} levels, renal and lipid status, and body mass index and assessing eating and fitness behaviors. Accordingly, it is best managed with ongoing specific measures of response to hypoglycemic agents and behavioral treatments, and by assessing an expanding array of risks and expected comorbid conditions, such as vascular conditions affecting the eyes, the skin, and elsewhere based on disease progression. Similarly, hyperlipidemia is diagnosed and managed with ongoing laboratory measurements and behavioral assessments, and treatment is directed toward not only the elevated lab value but also risks to other body systems. Management of chronic lung, kidney, and rheumatologic diseases similarly measures many domains of body function over time. Chronic disease management also requires "system-based" care, involving collaborative systems between patient, physician and nursing and other disciplines.[1-4] Focusing on just the patient complaint ("polydipsia") or laboratory result ("high cholesterol") does not meet current standard-of-care practices. Treatment of complex chronic illness requires ongoing assessments of many domains and adjustments to care based on how the patient responds to interventions prescribed or otherwise recommended.

Diagnosing and Managing a Difficult Pain Problem

Chronic pain is a complex disorder, much like any other chronic medical illness. It is commonly encountered in primary care practice, although chronic pain management is rarely taught at either the undergraduate or postgraduate level.[5-7] Chronic pain is nearly always a multisystem disorder, affecting both peripheral tissues and the central nervous system neuroplastic physiologic response (chronicization, or central sensitization),[8] as well as behavioral propensities and reactions to the diagnosed condition. Chronic pain is best understood to be a complex primary care condition requiring use of measurement-based tools and treatment algorithms so essential to the care and management of similar primary care conditions. Pain specialists have a consultative role, with occasional utility for procedural, behavioral, and rehabilitative intervention, but long-term oversight and continued treatment of pain always reside with the primary care physician.

Measurement-Based Tools to Assess Chronic Pain

John Bonica's 1954 identification of the need for psychiatrists in the treatment of chronic pain and Wilbur Fordyce's 1968 recognition of specific learned behaviors affecting treatment of chronic pain led quickly to the introduction of psychological measures to assess chronic pain.[9,10] The McGill Pain Questionnaire (MPQ) (Fig. 11.1) and the Minnesota Multiphasic Personality Inventory (MMPI) soon became widely used measurement tools in chronic pain treatment.[11–15] The MPQ was later shortened to the SF-MPQ (Fig. 11.2) and has since been validated as a measure to detect differences between various pain treatment effects.[16] Measuring patient function was introduced by Cleeland and his group using the Wisconsin Brief Pain Questionnaire (BPQ), recognizing the importance of pain interference with patient activity, and later revised for cancer pain as the Brief Pain Inventory (BPI) that was subsequently validated for noncancer chronic pain[17–19] (Fig. 11.3). The BPI measures pain intensity and interference with seven domains of function: general activity, mood, walking ability, normal work, relations with other persons, sleep, and enjoyment of life on a 0 to 10 scale. Recently, Dworkin and others have recommended that six similar measures be considered core outcome considerations when assessing pain treatment efficacy in their IMMPACT report (Table 11.1).[20,21] Many other validated tools assessing function and mood are also available, including the Roland-Morris Disability Questionnaire (RMDQ) (Fig. 11.4) and Oswestry Disability Index (Fig. 11.5), and the Personal Health Questionnaire for depression (PHQ-9).[22–24] The PHQ-9 tool has been used in many clinical studies of chronic pain disorders.[25–28]

Various pain treatment guidelines have also been published identifying the need to widen the assessment of pain beyond measuring just its intensity, including physical and emotional functioning and treatment risks, especially regarding opioid use.[29–32] Washington State Department of Health quality assurance boards now mandate use of guidelines requiring measurement of pain and treatment risks when opioids are prescribed long term.[33] Measurement of substance abuse risk fits well within the IMMPACT "adherence to treatment" category.

The importance of assessing risk of substance abuse cannot be understated. All primary care physicians encounter this regularly, and in fact, medical students are reconsidering their initial intent to pursue primary care practice based on their observations of practice dissatisfaction based on this factor alone.[34] There are voluminous published reports of comorbid substance abuse among chronic

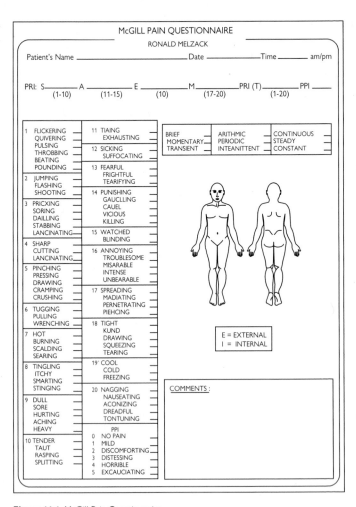

Figure 11.1 McGill Pain Questionnaire.

pain patients, with an incidence ranging from to 5% to 43%.[35–38] Considerable evidence also supports poor outcomes in pain treatment when addiction and psychiatric comorbidity are also present.[39,40] The highest-risk patients requesting the highest-risk treatments at the highest doses means that the highest level of precautions be followed. Recommended addiction assessment tools include the quickly administered 10-question Opioid Risk Tool (Fig. 11.6), the Screener and Opioid Assessment for Patients with Pain—Revised (SOAPP-R), or other structured interview approaches.[41–43]

Short-Form McGill Pain Questionnaire-2 (SF-MPQ-2)

This questionnaire provides you with a list of words that describe some of the different qualities of pain and related symptoms. Please put an X through the numbers that best describe the intensity of each of the pain and related symptoms you felt during the past week. Use 0 if the word does not describe your pain or related symptoms.

1. Throbbing pain	none	0	1	2	3	4	5	6	7	8	9	10	worst possible
2. Shooting pain	none	0	1	2	3	4	5	6	7	8	9	10	worst possible
3. Stabbing pain	none	0	1	2	3	4	5	6	7	8	9	10	worst possible
4. Sharp pain	none	0	1	2	3	4	5	6	7	8	9	10	worst possible
5. Cramping pain	none	0	1	2	3	4	5	6	7	8	9	10	worst possible
6. Gnawing pain	none	0	1	2	3	4	5	6	7	8	9	10	worst possible
7. Hot-burning pain	none	0	1	2	3	4	5	6	7	8	9	10	worst possible
8. Aching pain	none	0	1	2	3	4	5	6	7	8	9	10	worst possible
9. Heavy pain	none	0	1	2	3	4	5	6	7	8	9	10	worst possible
10. Tender	none	0	1	2	3	4	5	6	7	8	9	10	worst possible
11. Splitting pain	none	0	1	2	3	4	5	6	7	8	9	10	worst possible
12. Tiring-exhausting	none	0	1	2	3	4	5	6	7	8	9	10	worst possible
13. Sickening	none	0	1	2	3	4	5	6	7	8	9	10	worst possible
14. Fearful	none	0	1	2	3	4	5	6	7	8	9	10	worst possible
15. Punishing-cruel	none	0	1	2	3	4	5	6	7	8	9	10	worst possible
16. Electric-shock pain	none	0	1	2	3	4	5	6	7	8	9	10	worst possible
17. Cold-freezing pain	none	0	1	2	3	4	5	6	7	8	9	10	worst possible
18. Piercing	none	0	1	2	3	4	5	6	7	8	9	10	worst possible
19. Pain caused by light touch	none	0	1	2	3	4	5	6	7	8	9	10	worst possible
20. Itching	none	0	1	2	3	4	5	6	7	8	9	10	worst possible
21. Tingling or 'pins and needles'	none	0	1	2	3	4	5	6	7	8	9	10	worst possible
22. Numbness	none	0	1	2	3	4	5	6	7	8	9	10	worst possible

©R. Melzack and the Initiative on Methods, Measurement, and Pain Assessment in Clinical Trials (IMMP ACT). Information regarding permission to reproduce the SF- MPQ-2 can be obtained at www.immpact.org.

Figure 11.2 Short-Form McGill Pain Questionnaire-2.

Recently available public (National Institute of Health-PROMIS) domains and several commercial products are grouping together separate multidimensional testing instruments including pain, function, mood, quality of life, global improvement, and addiction risk.[44–47] These instruments are useful for primary care and specialty clinicians, facilitating the evaluation of many domains of pain simultaneously over the extended time for clinically important longitudinal treatment.

Measurement of chronic pain across many domains is crucial when assessing pain, selecting appropriate pain treatment, and following outcome of treatments prescribed. Pain intensity, while a critical fifth vital sign for "acute" pain,

STUDY ID# _____   HOSPITAL # _____
                        DO NOT WRITE ABOVE THIS LINE
                      Brief Pain Inventory (Short Form)

Date: ____/____/____   Time: _____
Name: _____
                    Last   First   Middle Initail

1. Thoughout our lives, most of us have had pain from time to time (such as minor
    headaches, sprains, and toothaches). Have you had pain other then these every-
    day kinds of pain today?

                    1.   Yes   2.   No

2. On the diagram, shade in the areas where you feel pain. Put and X on the area that
    hurts the most

3. Please rate your pain by circling the one number that best describes your pain at its
    worst in the last 24 hours.

    0   1   2   3   4   5   6   7   8   9   10
    No   Pain as bad as
    Pain   you can imagine

4. Please rate your pain by circling the one number that best describes your pain at its
    least in the last 24 hours.

    0   1   2   3   4   5   6   7   8   9   10
    No   Pain as bad as
    Pain   you can imagine

5. Please rate your pain by circling the one number that best describes your pain on
    the average

    0   1   2   3   4   5   6   7   8   9   10
    No   Pain as bad as
    Pain   you can imagine

6. Please rate your pain by circling the one number that tells how much pain you have
    right now.

    0   1   2   3   4   5   6   7   8   9   10
    No   Pain as bad as
    Pain   you can imagine

7. What treatments or medications are you recieving for your pain?

_____

8. In the last 24 hours, how much relief have pain treatments or medications
    provided? Please circle the one percentage that most shows how much relief
    you have received.

    0%   10% 20% 30% 40% 50% 60% 70% 80% 90% 100%
    No   Complete
    Relief   Relief

Figure 11.3 Brief Pain Inventory (Short Form).

9. Circle the one number that describes how, during the past 24 hours, pain has interfered with your:

A.   General Activity

0	1	2	3	4	5	6	7	8	9	10

Does not
Interfere   Completely
                                                                                 Interferes

B.   Mood

0	1	2	3	4	5	6	7	8	9	10

Does not
Interfere   Completely
                                                                                 Interferes

C.   Walking Ability

0	1	2	3	4	5	6	7	8	9	10

Does not
Interfere   Completely
                                                                                 Interferes

D.   Normal Work (includes both work outside the home and housework)

0	1	2	3	4	5	6	7	8	9	10

Does not
Interfere   Completely
                                                                                 Interferes

E.   Relations with other people

0	1	2	3	4	5	6	7	8	9	10

Does not
Interfere   Completely
                                                                                 Interferes

F.   Sleep

0	1	2	3	4	5	6	7	8	9	10

Does not
Interfere   Completely
                                                                                 Interferes

G.   Enjoyment of life

0	1	2	3	4	5	6	7	8	9	10

Does not
Interfere   Completely
                                                                                 Interferes

Figure 11.3 (continued)

Table 11.1 Core Domains for Clinical Trials of Chronic Pain Treatment Efficacy and Effectiveness

Pain

Physical functioning

Emotional functioning

Participant ratings of global improvement

Symptoms and adverse events

Participant disposition (including adherence to the treatment regimen and reasons for premature withdrawal from the trial)

From Turk DC, Dworkin RH, Allen RR, et al., Core outcome domains for chronic pain clinical trials: IMMPACT recommendations. *Pain.* 2003;106:337–345.

Patient name: _____ File # _____ Date: _____
Please read instructions: When your back hurts, you may find it difficult to do some of the things you normally do. Mark only the sentences that describe you today

☐ I stay at home most of the time because of my back.
☐ I change position frequently to try to get my back comfortable.
☐ I walk more slowly than usual because of my back.
☐ Because of my back, I am not doing any jobs that usually do around the house.
☐ Because of my back, I use a handrail to get upstairs.
☐ Because of my back, I lie down to rest more often.
☐ Because of my back, I have to hold on to something to get out of an easy chair.
☐ Because of my back, I try to get other people to do things for me.
☐ I get dressed more slowly than usual because of my back.
☐ I only stand up for short periods of time because of my back.
☐ Because of my back, I try not to bend or kneel down.
☐ I find it difficult to get out of a chair because of my back.
☐ My back is painful almost all of the time.
☐ I find it difficult to turn over in bed because of my back.
☐ My appetite is not very good because of my back.
☐ I have trouble putting on my sock (or stockings) because of the pain in my back.
☐ I can only walk short distances because of my back pain.
☐ I sleep less well because of my back.
☐ Because of my back pain, I get dressed with the help of someone else.
☐ I sit down for most of the day because of my back.
☐ I avoid heavy jobs around the house because of my back.
☐ Because of back pain, I am more irritable and bad tempered with people than usual.
☐ Because of back, I go upstairs more slowly than usual.
☐ I stay in bed most of the time because of my back.

Figure 11.4 Roland-Morris Disability Questionnaire.

is not useful as a single measure for "chronic" pain disorders. Chronic pain is a complex disease and, like the other chronic medical disorders managed by primary care physicians, requires an ongoing multidimensional assessment.

Use and Interpretation of Specific Measurements of Pain in This Case

Comprehensive assessment of Alice's persistent pain was extremely informative and redirected her care. Previous record review had documented only her subjective report of pain intensity; it showed that her pain ranged between 4 and 6/10 initially and then between 8 and 10/10 before and after each surgical and medical treatment. Her physical function demonstrated progressive deterioration and worsened after each surgical and medical intervention; she was painfully self-catheterizing 4 times a day, had voluntarily relinquished care of her young children to her mother, and was unable to participate in any home chore or marital intimacy.

Alice was then evaluated across the six recommended pain treatment domains. Her *pain intensity* was 8/10 at baseline, ranging from 4/10 on her opioids and "12/10" with attempted sexual activity. From this it was evident that her pain medication use was associated with subjective improvement, and that sexual contact caused pain beyond the most extreme reportable. This off-the-scale pain intensity suggested that her degree of distress was beyond what this evaluator could even consider imaginable. Extremely "abnormal" measures should be explored further, rather than discounted.

Her *physical function* was measured with a RMDQ and her score was 24/24. This supported her profound disability in all aspects of her life. Many experts deploy the RMDQ for pain conditions other than just back pain. An Oswestry

Section 1: Pain Intensity

☐ I have no pain at the moment
☐ The pain is very mild at the moment
☐ The pain is moderate at the moment
☐ The pain is fairly severe at the moment
☐ The pain is very severe at the moment
☐ The pain is the worst imaginable at the moment

Section 2: Personal Care (eg. washing, dressing)

☐ I can look after myself normally without causing extra pain
☐ I can look after myself normally but it causes extra pain
☐ It is painful to look after myself and i am slow and careful
☐ I need some help but can manage most of my personal care
☐ I need help every say in most aspects of self-care
☐ I do not get dressed, wash with difficulty and stay in bed

Section 3: Lifting

☐ I can lift heavy weights without extra pain
☐ I can lift heavy weights but it gives me extra pain
☐ Pain prevents me lifting heavy weights off the floor but I can manage if they are conveniently placed eg. on a table
☐ Pain prevents me lifting heavy weights but I can manage light to medium weights if they are conveniently positioned
☐ I can only lift very light weights
☐ I cannot lift or carry anything

Section 4: Walking*

☐ Pain does not prevent me walking any distance
☐ Pain prevents me from walking more than 2 kilometers
☐ Pain prevents me from walking more than 1 kilometer
☐ Pain prevents me from walking more than 500 metres
☐ I can only walk using a stick or crutches
☐ I am in bed most of the time

Section 5: Sitting

☐ I can sit in any chair as long as I like
☐ I can only sit in my favourite chair as long as I like
☐ Pain prevents me sitting more than one hour
☐ Pain prevents me from sitting more than 30 minutes
☐ Pain prevents me from sitting more than 10 minutes
☐ Pain prevents me from sitting at all

Section 6: Standing

☐ I can stand as long as I want without extra pain
☐ I can stand as long as I want but it gives me extra pain
☐ Pain prevents me from standing for more than 1 hour
☐ Pain prevents me from standing for more than 30 minutes
☐ Pain prevents me from standing for more than 10 minutes
☐ Pain prevents me from standing at all

Section 7: Sleeping

☐ My sleep is never disturbed by pain
☐ My sleep is occasionally disturbed by pain
☐ Because of pain I have less than 6 hours sleep
☐ Because of pain I have less than 4 hours sleep
☐ Because of pain I have less than 2 hours sleep
☐ Pain prevents me from sleeping at all

Section 8: Sex Life (if applicable)

☐ My sex life is normal and causes no extra pain
☐ My sex life is normal but causes some extra pain
☐ My sex life is nearly normal but is very painful
☐ My sex life is severely restricted by pain
☐ My sex life is nearly absent because of pain
☐ Pain prevents any sex life at all

Section 9: Social Life

☐ My social life is normal and gives me no extra pain
☐ My social life is normal but increases the degree of pain
☐ Pain has no significant effect on my social life apart from limiting my more energetic interests e.g. sport
☐ Pain has restricted my social life and I do not go out as often
☐ Pain has restricted my social life to my home
☐ I have no social life because of pain

Section 10: Travelling

☐ I can travel anywhere without pain
☐ I can travel any where but it gives me extra pain
☐ Pain is bad but I manage journeys over two hours
☐ Pain restricts me to journeys of less than one hour
☐ Pain restricts me to short necessary journeys under 30 minutes
☐ Pain prevents me from travelling except to receive treatment

Figure 11.5 Oswestry Disability Index.

Disability Questionnaire would also have resulted in very high impairment, especially with its questions specifically directed at sexual function. As will be seen, Alice's personal history of repeated physical and sexual abuse is an important diagnostic and treatment issue.

Her *emotional functioning* was poor, as expected: a PHQ-9 score of 24/27 indicated severe depression, and a Generalized Anxiety Disorder-7 (GAD-7) score of 18/21 indicated severe anxiety. After the first visit, posttraumatic stress was assessed using a 17-item civilian posttraumatic stress disorder (PTSD) assessment tool, which took 4 minutes to complete, quickly confirming this diagnosis based on Alice's extremely elevated score of 50 (Fig. 11.7). Open-ended questioning directed toward her sexual abuse history yielded a tale of an alcoholic and pain-pill-taking father regularly beating her mother, then sexually abusing the patient before she was age 12, prompting her to escape into a marriage to an alcoholic and abusive husband. She avoided sex by using pregnancy as her

Physician Form
With Item Value to Determine Risk Score

Name _____   Date _____

Mark each box that applies		Female	Male
1. Family history of substance abuse	■ Alchohol ■ Illegal drugs ■ Prescription drugs	[ ] 1 [ ] 2 [ ] 4	[ ] 3 [ ] 3 [ ] 4
2. Personal history of substance abuse	■ Alchohol ■ Illegal drugs ■ Prescription drugs	[ ] 3 [ ] 4 [ ] 5	[ ] 3 [ ] 4 [ ] 5
3. Age (mark box if 16-45 years)		[ ] 1	[ ] 1
4. History of preadolescent sexual abuse		[ ] 3	[ ] 0
5. Psychological disease	■ Attention-deficit/ hyperactivity disorder, obsessive-compulsive disorder, bipolar disorder, schizophrenia ■ Depression	[ ] 2 [ ] 1	[ ] 2 [ ] 1
Low (0–3) Moderate (4–7) High (≥8)	**Scoring totals**	[ ]	[ ]

Figure 11.6 Opioid Risk Tool.

way to resist his demands. Following hysterectomy, pregnancy was "medically" impossible, so her refusal of sex enraged her husband to the point where he verbally and physically abused her.

Once Alice committed to focusing on managing her emotional factors rather than on the futile search for miracle treatments, she acknowledged that her status quo was poor. She had struggled with a profound and long-established belief that improvement was impossible as she was still reporting pain at 6 to 8/10, even after years of treatment. Alice's initial self-reported quality of life was recorded at 1/6, but after 12 weeks of treatment, she had a reported quality-of-life improvement to 3/6, identifying a 50% *self-rating of global improvement*. Showing her that 50% was a very dramatic objective measure of improvement convinced her that change was possible, and continued treatment success was reinforced. She remained engaged in care and now embraced a commitment to further change. The recorded improvement measures kept her motivated to persist during her difficult first few months of treatment.

She was initially reluctant to reduce opioids but tolerated dose reduction quite well. She did agree that opioid treatment and self-catheterization were producing *adverse effects of treatment*. Because she developed side effects to the tricyclic antidepressant drugs offered, including dry mouth and constipation, they were switched to a serotonin-norepinephrine receptor inhibitor (SNRI),

INSTRUCTIONS: Below is a list of problems and complaints that people sometimes have in response to stressful life experiences. Please read each one carefully, then circle one of the numbers to the right to indicate how much you have been bothered by that problem in the past month.

		Not at all	A little bit	Moderately	Quite a bit	Extremely
1.	Repeated, disturbing *memories, thoughts* or *images* of a stressful experience from the past?	1	2	3	4	5
2.	Repeated, disturbing *dreams* of a stressful experience from the past?	1	2	3	4	5
3.	Suddenly *acting* or *feeling* as if a stressfull experience were *happening again* (as if you were reliving it)?	1	2	3	4	5
4.	Feeling *very upset* when *something reminded you* of a stressful experience from the past?	1	2	3	4	5
5.	Having *physical reactions* (e.g., heart pounding, trouble breathing, sweating) when *something reminded you* of a stressful experience from the past?	1	2	3	4	5
6.	Avoiding *thinking about* or *talking about* a stressful experience from the past or avoiding *having feelings* related to it?	1	2	3	4	5
7.	Avoiding *activities or situations because they reminded you* of a stressful experience from the past?	1	2	3	4	5
8.	Trouble *remembering important parts* of a stressful experience from the past?	1	2	3	4	5
9.	*Loss of interest* in ativities that you used to enjoy?	1	2	3	4	5
10.	Feeling *distant* or *cut off* from other people?	1	2	3	4	5
11.	Feeling *emotionally numb* or being unable to have loving feelings for those close to you?	1	2	3	4	5
12.	Feelings as if your *future* will somehow be *cut short*?	1	2	3	4	5
13.	Trouble *falling or staying asleep*?	1	2	3	4	5
14.	Feeling *irritable* or having *angry outbursts*?	1	2	3	4	5
15.	Having *difficulty concentrating*?	1	2	3	4	5
16.	Being " *super-alert*" or watchful or on guard?	1	2	3	4	5
17.	Feeling *jumpy* or easily startled?	1	2	3	4	5

Figure 11.7 Civilian PTSD Check List (PCL-C).

and she was satisfied that the new approach were far less adverse than her prior treatments.

Based on the initial high score of 13 on her Opioid Risk Tool, it was not surprising that she had previously misused her opioid prescriptions. Tapering doses to get her off opioids was supported by regular urine drug testing, confirming *treatment adherence*. She failed to keep her initial cognitive behavioral psychotherapy sessions, but after she was specifically informed that participation *in all aspects* of her recommended care was also considered a crucially important component of treatment compliance, she attended all subsequent sessions. Seeing her progress, she quickly accepted a nonopioid pain plan, and in fact admitted herself into an intensive substance use facility for "after-care" even after she was long off opioids.

This case illustrates the power of measurement and data in managing complex pain. In Alice's case, comprehensive measurements of mood, abuse history, function, and quality of life had either not been taken or not used as a focus for treatment. It is increasingly recognized that the physical manifestation of pain may reflect underlying psychic distress, which if addressed may improve pain and reduce reliance on drugs and injections. In this patient's case, being able to see the trends in her own self-reports was valuable because it allowed her to understand how her pain could be influenced through attention to underlying factors. It also helped her understand how much more effective her new control strategies were compared with her prior focus on surgical procedures and medications. Estimated total time to take all the aforementioned recommended initial tests is less than 10 minutes: **pain intensity**, less than 30 seconds; **physical function** using Roland-Morris or Oswestry, approximately 3 minutes; **emotional function** using PHQ-9, less than 1 minute (later PTSD testing, ≤5 minutes); **global quality of life**, less than 30 seconds; and **Opioid Risk Tool**, less than or equal to 2 minutes. Had these been assessed earlier, Alice's care may have been different. The initial assessment may have revealed the deep-rooted psychological distress underlying her pain, allowing for early intervention. Subsequent measures and trends may have revealed much sooner the limited role of surgical intervention and medication and prevented futile dose escalation. Early and continuous measurement in this case would have likely saved time, trauma, and expense.

Ethical Issues When Complex Pain Assessment and Outcomes Are Not Measured

Pelvic pain is by no means easy for the patient to live with or for the doctor to assess and treat properly. In Alice's case it was complicated at the outset by her pregnancy, and soon after when endometriosis was visualized. However, after treatment of endometriosis, her pain not only persisted but also worsened. Published reports and meta-analyses assessing outcomes of surgical, medical, and multidisciplinary treatments support early diagnosis and treatment of surgical disease, such as endometriosis or when there is evidence of high-grade adhesions causing bowel obstruction; but, absent-well defined pathoanatomy, evidence favors multidisciplinary nonsurgical management.[48] Certainly Alice's history of sexual abuse and its complex consequences in her life, which she stated *had never been asked about* prior, were obviously quite important. She underwent increasingly extensive gynecologic surgery, then increasingly invasive urologic treatments without evident improvement. She was treated with escalating doses of opioids, sedatives, and hypnotics with no record of effect except, "I think they lessen my pain (intensity)." An alternative diagnosis could have been made far earlier had her abuse history been taken; the Opioid Risk Tool would have prompted a differential diagnosis directed toward psychosocial distress, not a urogynecologic entity that could be removed or manipulated. The ethical dilemma here is not which specialty is responsible for making the correct diagnosis, but rather how to reduce harm to a woman seeking a cure to a mysterious painful disorder. Harm can be reduced when physicians follow diagnostic and treatment approaches appropriate to the presenting complaint. Complex chronic pain requires diagnosis and management consistent with any complex chronic disorder.

Summary Points: Care Recommendations Based on Measurement-Based Tools

Alice was treated for her depression with tricyclic antidepressants and later SNRI antidepressants. Her PTSD was treated with prazosin. Her sedative drugs (carisoprodol and alprazolam) were slowly withdrawn. She was referred for cognitive behavioral therapy to address her PTSD and mood response to her catastrophic early and adult life abuse experiences. She was taken off her long-acting opioid (OxyContin) and provided with decreasing doses of hydrocodone until she was off opioids entirely. She participated in an outpatient women's 12-step support group. She filed for divorce and her husband moved out of her home. She began to coparent with her mother, who also began supportive counseling to address her own despair and distress regarding the terrible family circumstances in which she passively participated. For Alice, 10 minutes of measurement time could have directed treatment more appropriately, avoided multiple ineffective procedures, and prevented years of overreliance on opioids.

References

1. Hassey A. Complexity in the clinical encounter. In: Sweeny K, Griffiths F, eds. *Complexity and healthcare*. Radcliffe Medical Press, Oxon OX. 2002:60–73.

2. Greenhalgh T. Narrative based medicine in an evidence based world. *BMJ*. 1999;318:323–325.

3. Von Korff M, Gruman J, Schaefer J, Curry SJ, Wagner EH. Collaborative management of chronic illness. *Ann Intern Med*. 1997;127:1097–1102.

4. Strange KC, Nutting PA, Miller WL, et al. Defining and measuring the patient-centered medical home. *J Gen Intern Med*. 2010;25:601–612.

5. Briggs EV, Carr E, Whittaker MS. Survey of undergraduate pain curricula for healthcare professionals in the United Kingdom. *Eur J Pain*. 2011;15:789–795.

6. Mezei L, Murinson BB: Pain education in North American medical schools. *J Pain* 2011; 424(12):1199–1208..

7. Bair MJ. Learning from our learners: implications for pain management education in medical schools. *Pain Med*. 2011;12:1139–1141.

8. Woolf CJ. Central sensitization: implications for the diagnosis and treatment of pain. *Pain*. 2011;152(3 Suppl):S2–S15.

9. Bonica JJ. The role of the anesthetist in the management of intractable pain. *Proc Royal Soc Med*. 1954;47:1029–1032.

10. Fordyce WE, Fowler RS, Lehman JF, DeLatour B. Some implications of learning in problems of chronic pain. *J Chronic Dis*. 1968;21:179–190.

11. Melzack R. The McGill Pain Questionnaire: major properties and scoring methods. *Pain.* 1975;1:277–299.

12. Roberts AH, Reinhardt L. The behavioral management of chronic pain: long-term follow-up with comparison groups. *Pain.* 1980;8:151–162.

13. McGill JC, Lawlis GF, Selby D, Mooney V, McCoy CE. The relationship of Minnesota Multiphasic Personality Inventory (MMPI) profile clusters to pain behaviors. *J Behav Med.* 1983;6:77–92.

14. Love AW, Peck CL. The MMPI and psychological factors in chronic low back pain: a review. *Pain.* 1987;28:1–12.

15. Swimmer GI, Robinson ME, Geisser ME. Relationship of MMPI cluster type, pain coping strategy, and treatment outcome. *Clin J Pain.* 1992;8:131–137.

16. Dworkin RH, Turk DC, Revicki DA, et al. Development and initial validation of an expanded and revised version of the Short-form McGill Pain Questionnaire (SF-MPQ-2). *Pain.* 2009;144:35–42.

17. Daut RL, Cleeland CS, Flanery RC. Development of the Wisconsin Brief Pain Questionnaire to assess pain in cancer and other diseases. *Pain.* 1983;17:197–210.

18. Cleeland CS. Measurement of pain by subjective report. In: Chapman CR, Loeser JD, eds. *Advances in pain research and therapy. Vol. 12. Issues in Pain Measurement.* New York: Raven Press; 1989:391–403.

19. Tan G, Jensen MP, Thornby JI, Shanti BF. Validation of the Brief Pain Inventory for chronic nonmalignant pain. *J Pain.* 2004;5:133–137.

20. Turk DC, Dworkin RH, Allen RR, et al. Core outcome domains for chronic pain clinical trials: IMMPACT recommendations. *Pain.* 2003;106:337–345.

21. Dworkin RH, Turk DC, McDermott MP, et al. Interpreting the clinical importance of group differences in chronic pain clinical trials: IMMPACT recommendations. *Pain.* 2009;146:238–244.

22. Roland M, Fairbank J. The Roland-Morris Disability Questionnaire and the Oswestry Disability Questionnaire. *Spine.* 2000;25:3115–3124.

23. Cleland J, Gillani R, Bienen EJ, Sadosky A. Assessing dimensionality and responsiveness of outcomes measures for patients with low back pain. *Pain Pract.* 2010;11:57–69.

24. Kroenke K, Spitzer RL, Williams J, Lowe B. The patient health questionnaire somatic, anxiety, and depressive symptom scales: a systematic review. *Gen Hosp Psychiatry.* 2010;32:345–359.

25. Turner JA, Dworkin SF. Screening for psychosocial risk factors in patients with chronic orofacial pain—recent advances. *J Am Dent Assoc.* 2004;135:1119–1125.

26. Gameroff MJ, Olfson M. Major depressive disorder, somatic pain, and health care costs in an urban primary care practice. *J Clin Psychiatry.* 2006;67:1232–1239.

27. Kroenke K, Bair M, Damush T, et al. Stepped care for affective disorders and musculoskeletal pain (SCAMP) study design and practical implications of an intervention for comorbid pain and depression. *Gen Hosp Psychiatry.* 2007;29:506–517.

28. Dobscha SK, Corson K, Perrin NA, et al. Collaborative care for chronic pain in primary care: a clustered randomized trial. *JAMA.* 2009;301:1242–1252.

29. Washington State Agency Medical Director Group. *Interagency guideline on opioid dosing for chronic non-cancer pain.* 2010. http://www.agencymeddirectors. wa.gov/opioiddosing.asp (accessed November 26, 2011).

30. Rolfs RT, Johnson E, Williams NJ, Sundwall DN, Utah guidelines on pre-scribing opioids for treatment of pain. *J Pain Palliat Care Pharmacother.* 2010;24:219–235.

31. Furlan AD, Reardon R, Weppler C. Opioids for chronic noncancer pain: a new Canadian practice guideline. *CMAJ.* 2010;182:923–930.

32. National Guideline Clearinghouse, Agency for Healthcare Research and Quality, US Department of Health and Human Services. http://www.guideline. gov/search/search.aspx?term=chronic+pain (accessed November 26, 2011).

33. Washington State Department of Health. http://www.doh.wa.gov/hsqa/profes-sions/painmanagement/ (accessed November 26, 2011).

34. Corrigan C, Desnick L, Marshall S, Bentov N, Rosenblatt R. What can we learn from first-year medical students' perceptions of pain in the primary care setting? *Pain Med.* 2011;12:1216–1222.

35. Martells BA, O'Connor PG, Kerns RD, et al. Systematic review: opioid treat-ment for chronic low back pain: prevalence, efficacy, and association with addic-tion. *Ann Intern Med.* 2007;146:116–127.

36. Ives TJ., Chelmínski PR., Hammett-Stable CA, etal., Opioid misuse in patients with chronic pain: a prospective cohortstudy. *BMC Health Serv Res;* 2006,6:46–56

37. Ballantyne JC, LaForge SL. Opioid dependenceand addiction in opioid treated pain patients. Pain 2007;129:235–55.

38. FlemingMF, Balousek SL, Klessig CL, Mundt MP, Brown DD. Substance use disorders in a primary care sample receiving daily opioid therapy. *J Pain.* 2007;8:573–582

39. Morasco BJ, Corson K, Turk DC, Dobscha SK. Association between substance use disorder status and pain-related function following 12 months of treatment in primary care patients with musculoskeletal pain. *J Pain.* 2011;12:352–359.

40. Pignone MP. A primary care, multi-disciplinary disease management program for opioid-treated patients with chronic non-cancer pain and a high burden of psychiatric comorbidity. *BMC Health Serv Res.* 2005;5:3.

41. Webster LR, Webster RM. Predicting aberrant behaviors in opioid-treated patients: preliminary validation of the opioid risk tool. *Pain Med.* 2005;6(6):432–442.

42. Savage SR. Assessment for addiction in pain-treatment settings. *Clin J Pain.* 2002;18(Suppl 4):S28–S38.

43. Fine PG, Finnegan T, Portenoy RK. Protect your patients-protect your practice: practical risk assessment in the structuring of opioid therapy in chronic pain. *J Fam Pract.* 2010;59(Suppl 2):S1–S16.

44. NIH's Patient Reported Outcomes Measurement Information System (PROMIS). http://www.nihpromis.org/ (accessed November 27, 2011).

45. CPAIN—Registrat-MAPI. http://www.cpain.com (accessed November 27, 2011).

46. PRISM—ProCare Systems Pain Evaluations Tool—Dynamic Clinical Systems. http://www.procareresearch.com/services_prism.html (accessed November 27, 2011).

47. POET (Pain Outcomes Evaluation Tool)—Dynamic Clinical Systems. http://dynamicclinical.com (accessed November 27, 2011).

48. Stones W, Cheong YC, Howard FM, Singh S. Interventions for treating chronic pelvic pain in women. *Cochrane Database Syst Rev.* 2005;(2):CD000387. doi:10.1002/14651858.C-000387

Chapter 12

Not a Suitable Candidate: Saying No

Jane C. Ballantyne

The Case

Joe Savor is a 33-year-old plumber who was in his usual state of health until he injured himself at work falling off a ladder. The fall resulted in a back injury with intense axial lower back pain with radiation down the left-leg lateral aspect and into the dorsum of the left foot. Because there were physical findings suggestive of radiculopathy, magnetic resonance imaging (MRI) was conducted, which revealed a disc protrusion at L4-L5. The decision was made to proceed with nonsurgical management consisting of physical therapy, epidural steroid injection, and opioids. The patient's radiculopathy improved, but after 6 weeks of attempted rehabilitation, he was still complaining of 9/10 axial low back pain with radiation to the left leg. He is able to ambulate but uses a cane. He does not feel able to return to work and is applying for disability.

Past medical history is notable only for steady alcohol use (two beers per night), smoking (one pack per day), teenage marijuana use, although none recently, and borderline hypertension (untreated). Family history is positive for alcoholism (father) and cancer (mother). The patient lives with his wife and two preadolescent children. His wife works as a floor manager for a large retail store.

Three months after the initial injury, Mr. Savor is referred to the pain clinic by his primary care physician because his pain, mobility, and function have not improved, and he is now taking opioids around the clock at a high dose. His pain treatment regimen consists of oxycodone 40 mg extended release 3 times daily with oxycodone 10 mg intermediate release up to 8 times daily. No other medications are prescribed.

List of Considerations

- At 3 months, pain is chronic and no longer subacute.
- At this point, a decision must be made about whether to continue opioid therapy as chronic opioid therapy (COT).

- Considering that prolonged opioid therapy (>3 months) typically becomes self-perpetuating and lifelong, this is the point at which an analysis should be made concerning benefits versus risks of COT for this patient.

Clinical Discussion

This is a patient who, within a short time frame (3 months) and after an ordinarily self-limited injury, is in danger of become chronically disabled by pain. Two issues arise:

1. What is the best way to treat his pain and restore his function at this 3-month point?
2. What is the role of opioids in his future pain management?

Treating Early-Onset Chronic Pain

One must first consider why Mr. Savor has persistent pain, when many patients with similar injuries might have achieved a complete recovery. The majority of patients treated for acute and subacute pain will recover normal or near-normal function, while choosing to end all pain medications.[1] When presented with a patient who does not recover as expected, it is always worth probing into possible motivators for prolonged disability and continued medication use. Often, chronic pain and disability develop in patients with mental health and substance abuse comorbidities, particularly posttraumatic stress disorder (PTSD).[2–6] In Mr. Savor's case, there is no history of mental health disorder, serious past substance abuse, or PTSD, although there is a family history of substance abuse (alcoholism). Further questioning could reveal active depression and anxiety, which is worth eliciting because treatment of depression and anxiety is often helpful when managing pain.[7,8] Work dissatisfaction can be a powerful factor in the secondary gain from prolonged pain and disability[9,10] and may be a factor in this patient. Discussion about work satisfaction, employment goals and lessening possible anticipatory fear of workplace reinjury can be another important avenue toward motivating patients like Mr. Savor to improve.

Once the difficult conversations have been had about underlying factors that could explain pain persistence, it becomes clearer what treatments should now be instituted to try to prevent pain chronicity. Motivational approaches would include, importantly, return to measured physical therapy and strengthening to prevent deconditioning. For depression and anxiety, if found, pharmacologic intervention and counseling can be helpful. Vocational counseling can also be enormously helpful if fear of returning to work is part of the developing disability syndrome. Nonopioid analgesics are notably absent from the patient's current medication regimen, and adjuncts such as acetaminophen, nonsteroidal anti-inflammatory drugs (NSAIDs), anticonvulsants, and antidepressants should be considered. It is always worth encouraging patients to pursue complementary or other nonmedical approaches such as acupuncture, aqua-therapy, tai chi, and massage.[11–13]

Role of Opioids in Long-Term Pain Management

Increasingly, population data suggest that chronic opioid therapy fails many patients in many senses. Safety issues aside, the treatment is not actually providing the pain relief expected on the basis of initial efficacy, and the idea that the development of tolerance that reduces analgesic efficacy can be overcome by open-ended dose escalation has largely been discredited.[14,15] The vast majority of patients taking long-term opioids report high pain scores, even after repeated dose escalation.[16–20] Doses can reach toxic levels, to the point that a hyperalgesic state develops, and to the point of opioid refractoriness, where patients become less sensitive to opioid treatment, should new pain arise.[21–23] Data on function and quality of life for patients on COT are less certain, yet some studies suggest actual functional deterioration with COT.[24–26] Does this mean that chronic pain patients are not being helped by opioids? One must remain open to the possibility that COT helps certain patients; especially considering that many patients, and their physicians,claim that their lives would be considerably worse without COT. One can posit a number of reasons that COT might relieve suffering in certain patients, including that the "numbing" effect of opioids is helpful for individuals with extreme existential suffering (a population that does indeed tend to end up on COT), and that for individuals with multiple drug sensitivities (e.g., the elderly), small doses of opioids taken occasionally can relieve pain.[20,27] Is the goal of COT to provide comfort, in the sense of palliation, or to achieve functional restoration?

When faced with any individual patient and the decision to embark on COT (or prolong opioid therapy beyond its acute or subacute phase), it is of paramount importance to establish the goal for this therapy. Mr. Savor is a young patient who, before he was injured was fully functional. While it is possible that since being injured, factors that could contribute to progression into a chronic pain state (e.g., work dissatisfaction, mental health or substance abuse disorder) could have been unmasked, it would seem important to establish with him a goal of returning to full functional capacity. Encouraging a belief that full-function restoration (or a least restoration appropriate to age and physical status) is possible is a vital part of the therapeutic interaction.

After establishing a goal of functional restoration, the decision to wean off opioids emerges as the correct decision. This is on the basis of strong evidence that COT is not effective at restoring function and may actually run counter to the goal of functional restoration because COT, through multiple mechanisms, promotes rest, not activity.[15,28] Among such mechanisms are effects on the hypothalamic-pituitary-adrenal axis, which produces hypogonadism; loss of libido, energy and drive; and infertility.[29–31]

The main argument for discontinuing opioid therapy in this patient centers on the knowledge that this therapy will not reduce pain to any useful degree over the long term and will not achieve the goal of functional restoration. Remembering that continued COT becomes self-perpetuating and potentially lifelong, the 3-month time point is a good opportunity to evaluate and reconsider. The risk of COT should also be considered, although this patient presents with few risk factors other than young age and possible substance abuse (alcohol, smoking).

Ethical Issues

Modern medical ethics focuses on the patient's right to determine treatment choices. The more traditional Hippocratic model whereby the physician healer was responsible for protecting the patient (doing no harm)—the paternalistic model of care—has long since given way to a guidance-cooperation model whereby the physician healer can advise but not determine medical decisions.[32,33] This is especially important in complex chronic illness management, and introduction of shared medical decision making in the management of chronic pain is expected to improve patient and provider satisfaction and other pain management outcomes.[34,35] The modern patient has autonomy and the right to choose or reject treatment.[36] Patient bills of rights advocate for patient choice, while declarations such as the pain charter and the more recent Montreal pain declaration present pain relief as a basic human right.[37–40] Read further into these mandates, and one could argue that when opioids are demanded, they should be provided. Pain is an experience that only a patient can know, so the treating clinician must rely on the patient's report. How, then, can one ever deny a patient opioid treatment if it is sought?

Return now to the basis of modern ethical decision making, the guidance-cooperation model. Within this model, the ideal would be that when the benefits and risks of a treatment are laid out logically by the better-informed and more experienced clinician, the patient will understand and agree with the clinician's assessment. In Mr. Savor's case, once the goals of treatment are established, the clinician can show that evidence and experience indicate that COT does not generally help toward the goal of functional restoration and produces only limited gains in terms of pain relief. Moreover, opioids produce dependence, and this phenomenon makes it hard to discontinue COT even in the face of poor outcome.[41] Ideally Mr. Savor understands and agrees.

The more difficult ethical dilemma arises when the prescriber does not want to prescribe but cannot convince the patient to accept the reasons for withholding treatment. So arises one of the most troubling ethical issues in modern medicine, which concerns the clinician's responsibility toward the individual patient, weighed against responsibility to society.[42] Traditionally it is politicians and regulators who have responsibility for society, while clinicians have primary responsibility for their patients. Thus, if prescribing harms society, in this case because it potentially enables a young patient to avoid the workplace, but satisfies the individual (who is unwilling to give up opioids), continued prescribing may be seen as ethically correct despite the potential harm to society. At the same time, there is also a principle that states that if the clinician perceives harm, there is no obligation to treat, and no obligation means there is no correlative right on the part of the patient.[43] This is the principle of correlativity, which states that a patient has no right to a treatment that a clinician feels under no obligation to provide. By this argument, because the clinician believes that opioid treatment will ultimately harm the patient, it would be ethical to withhold treatment without the patient's approval.

Initial Recommendations

Despite aggressive early attempts at rehabilitation, Mr. Savor presents 3 months after injury still out of work and still on opioid therapy. Pain after injury that persists up to 3 months is generally considered acute or subacute. Pain that persists after 3 months, or beyond the point where healing should be complete or near complete, is generally considered chronic. This is a useful point at which to reevaluate and come up with a new treatment plan. Unfortunately, it is all too common that opioid treatment of acute or sub-acute pain develops into COT through default, and not through deliberate thoughtful planning, the result being that patients are treated with COT who would have been selected out by a rational selection process. In Mr. Savor's case, avoiding COT will avoid putting him in the position of many other patients who function poorly on opioids but later find it hard to come off. For Mr. Savor, the initial treatment approach could be summarized as follows:

1. Establish pain treatment goals. Involve family in this whenever possible.
2. Encourage slow increase in physical activity and strength, preferably with the help of an expert physical therapist, to reverse and avoid future deconditioning.
3. Introduce adjuncts into the pharmacologic regimen.
4. Counsel, with emphasis on vocational counseling, toward a goal of return to appropriate work or activity, if not previous work.
5. Wean off opioids.
6. Encourage use of nonmedical approaches such as acupuncture, aquatherapy, tai chi, and massage.

Long-Term Plan

The initial recommendations all aim toward helping Mr. Savor avoid falling into the spiral of nonserious injury that escalates into chronic pain and disability, with chronicity being exacerbated and complicated by continued opioid therapy. An injury is often the trigger for the onset of age-related aches and pains, drastic changes in belief systems (concerning invulnerability), and loss of confidence. The constant plea of many such patients is, "I just want to be able to do what I used to be able to do." An important part of the clinician's role is to help the patient understand the power of self-management, the limitations of medical treatment (especially opioids), the inevitability of aging, and the ability of the human body to recover from injury—if not to an earlier age, then at least to an acceptable state compatible with age and injury status. Catastrophic thinking in terms of permanent disability, pain severe enough to warrant COT, and being in the sick role inevitably results in deteriorating health and quality of life. Mr. Savor's is a typical case where COT should be avoided: he is young and should not be started on a treatment that is likely to be lifelong and not produce gains in function; there is no clear etiology for his pain; and he needs to be motivated and activated, and opioids dampen motivation.

Summary Points

When is it appropriate to deny a patient opioid treatment? So much recent teaching suggests that we should never deny opioids to patients with stated pain, that opioids are needed because chronic pain is a growing problem, and that opioid intervention can reverse the problem of increasing pain prevalence.[39,44,45] Chronic pain is, indeed, increasing in prevalence as the population ages and as modern medicine makes disease and injury less rapidly fatal.[46] But we must seriously question whether opioids can reverse this trend. In fact, recent claims data strongly suggest that opioid management of chronic pain, while increasingly utilized, is producing a population of patients whose pain is not well controlled, whose function is poor, and who are suffering a number of adverse consequences of COT; including dependence and addiction, obstipation, poor sleep, worsened sleep apnea, loss of energy and drive, infertility, high fracture rates, and even drug-related death.[47–50] Much of this is related to high dose treatment, but data also show that patients who remain on opioids long term do tend to dose escalate, and for many of them, adverse effects predominate over any outcomes benefit.[2]

Mr. Savor presents as someone who could either become a chronically disabled patient whose pain and disability are validated and reinforced by continuing opioid treatment or become someone who could be motivated to achieve functional recovery, which would be aided by avoiding COT. In his case, it would seem both medically advisable and ethically justified to deny COT. Mr. Savor is one of many patients who currently fall into COT at a young age, without a firm pathoanatomic pain diagnosis, where COT contributes to worsening condition, function, and quality of life. In the opinion of this author, all young patients with pain that does not have a clear diagnosis should be denied COT.

There are other patients, however (not described in this chapter, which focuses on denying opioids), who likely do benefit from COT when carefully provided. They may be outnumbered, but there is a select group of patients who probably do benefit from COT, and many such cases are reviewed in other chapters in this book. We may be disillusioned about COT's ability to eradicate pain, but opioids can relieve complex suffering, and provided this treatment is reserved for patients whose suffering cannot be addressed in other ways, then it should be preserved. Hopefully we will not allow irrational prescribing and its disastrous adverse consequences to reduce availability for those in need. At heart, this chapter has been about reducing irrational prescribing so that opioids can be preserved for those who demonstrate benefit and who depend on opioids to make their lives tolerable.

References

1. Kalso E, Edwards J, Moore R, McQuay H. Opioids in chronic non-cancer pain: systematic review of efficacy and safety. *Pain*. 2004;112:372–380.

2. MartinBC, Fan MY, Edlund MJ, Devries A, Braden JB, Sullivan MD. Long-term chronic opioid therapy discontinuation rates from the TROUP study. *J Gen Intern Med*. 2011;26:1450–1457.

3. Sullivan MD. Who gets high-dose opioid therapy for chronic non-cancer pain? *Pain*. 2010;151:567–568.

4. Sullivan MD, Edlund MJ, Fan MY, Devries A, Brennan Braden J, Martin BC. Trends in use of opioids for non-cancer pain conditions 2000–2005 in commercial and Medicaid insurance plans: the TROUP study. *Pain*. 2008;138:440–449.

5. Boudreau D, Von Korff M, Rutter CM, et al. Trends in long-term opioid therapy for chronic non-cancer pain. *Pharmacoepidemiol Drug Saf*. 2009;18:1166–1175.

6. Edlund MJ, Martin BC, Devries A, Fan MY, Braden JB, Sullivan MD. Trends in use of opioids for chronic noncancer pain among individuals with mental health and substance use disorders: the TROUP study. *Clin J Pain*. 2010;26:1–8.

7. Bair MJ, Robinson RL, Katon W, Kroenke K. Depression and pain comorbidity: a literature review. *Arch Intern Med*. 2003;163:2433–2445.

8. Sullivan MJ, Reesor K, Mikail S, Fisher R. The treatment of depression in chronic low back pain: review and recommendations. *Pain*. 1992;50:5–13.

9. Krause N, Dasinger LK, Deegan LJ, Rudolph L, Brand RJ. Psychosocial job factors and return-to-work after compensated low back injury; a disability phase-specific analysis. *Am J Ind Med*. 2001;40:374–392.

10. Krause N, Frank JW, Dasinger LK, Sullivan TJ, Sinclair SJ. Determinants of duration of disability and return-to-work after work-related injury and illness: challenges for future research. *Am J Ind Med*. 2001;40:464–484.

11. Terhorst L, Schneider MJ, Kim KH, Goozdich LM, Stilley CS. Complementary and alternative medicine in the treatment of pain in fibromyalgia: a systematic review of randomized controlled trials. *J Manipulative Physiol Ther*. 2011;34:483–496.

12. Zhu X, Hamilton KD, McNicol ED. Acupuncture for pain in endometriosis. *Cochrane Database Syst Rev*. 2011;9:CD007864.

13. Posadzki P, Lizis P, Hagner-Derengowska M. Pilates for low back pain: a systematic review. *Complement Ther Clin Pract*. 2011;17:85–89.

14. Ballantyne JC, Shin NS. Efficacy of opioids for chronic pain: a review of the evidence. *Clin J Pain*. 2008;24:469–478.

15. Chou R, Fanciullo GJ, Fine PG, et al. Clinical guidelines for the use of chronic opioid therapy in chronic noncancer pain. *J Pain*. 2009;10:113–130.

16. Eriksen J, Sjogren P, Bruera E, Ekholm O, Rasmussen NK. Critical issues on opioids in chronic non-cancer pain. An epidemiological study. *Pain*. 2006;125:172–179.

17. Braden JB, Russo J, Fan MY, et al. Emergency department visits among recipients of chronic opioid therapy. *Arch Intern Med*. 2010;170:1425–1432.

18. Caudill-Slosberg M, Schwartz L, Woloshin S. Office visits and analgesic prescriptions for musculoskeletal pain in the US: 1980 vs 2000. *Pain*. 2004;109:524–529.

19. Dillie KS, Fleming MF, Mundt MP, French MT. Quality of life associated with daily opioid therapy in a primary care chronic pain sample. *J Am Board Fam Med*. 2008;21:108–117.

20. Wallace AS, Freburger JK, Darter JD, Jackman AM, Carey TS. Comfortably numb? Exploring satisfaction with chronic back pain visits. *Spine J.* 2009;9:721–728.

21. Angst MS, Clark JD. Opioid-induced hyperalgesia: a qualitative systematic review. *Anesthesiology.* 2006;104:570–587.

22. Chu LF, Angst MS, Clark D. Opioid-induced hyperalgesia in humans: molecular mechanisms and clinical considerations. *Clin J Pain.* 2008;24:479–496.

23. Devulder J. Hyperalgesia induced by high-dose intrathecal sufentanil in neuropathic pain. *J Neurosurg Anesthesiol.* 1997;9:146–148.

24. Turner JA, Franklin G, Fulton-Kehoe D, et al. ISSLS prize winner: early predictors of chronic work disability: a prospective, population-based study of workers with back injuries. *Spine (Phila Pa 1976).* 2008;33:2809–2818.

25. Franklin GM, Stover BD, Turner JA, Fulton-Kehoe D, Wickizer TM. Early opioid prescription and subsequent disability among workers with back injuries: the Disability Risk Identification Study Cohort. *Spine (Phila Pa 1976).* 2008;33:199–204.

26. Stover BD, Turner JA, Franklin G, et al. Factors associated with early opioid prescription among workers with low back injuries. *J Pain.* 2006;7:718–725.

27. Ballantyne JC. Patient-centered health care: are opioids a special case? *Spine J.* 2009;9:770–772.

28. Manchikanti L, Vallejo R, Manchikanti KN, Benyamin RM, Datta S, Christo PJ. Effectiveness of long-term opioid therapy for chronic non-cancer pain. *Pain Physician.* 2011;14:E133–E156.

29. Daniell HW. Hypogonadism in men consuming sustained-action oral opioids. *J Pain.* 2002;3:377–384.

30. Daniell HW. Narcotic-induced hypogonadism during therapy for heroin addiction. *J Addict Dis.* 2002;21:47–53.

31. Finch PM, Roberts LJ, Price L, Hadlow NC, Pullan PT. Hypogonadism in patients treated with intrathecal morphine. *Clin J Pain.* 2000;3:251–254.

32. Brennan TA. *Just doctoring. Medical ethics in the liberal state.* Berkeley and Los Angeles, CA: University of California Press; 1991:3 (Brennan quotes the Webster Dictionary definition of liberalism).

33. Szasz T, Hollender J. The basic model of the doctor-patients relationship. *Arch Int Med.* 1956;97:85–90.

34. Von Korff M, Gruman J, Schaefer J, Curry SJ, Wagner EH. Collaborative management of chronic illness. *Ann Intern Med.* 1997;127:1097–1102.

35.. Frantsve LM, Kerns RD. Patient-provider interactions in the management of chronic pain: current findings within the context of shared medical decision making. *Pain Med.* 2007;8:25–35.

36.. Barry MJ, Fowler FJ Jr, Mulley AG Jr, Henderson JV Jr, Wennberg JE. Patient reactions to a program designed to facilitate patient participation in treatment decisions for benign prostatic hyperplasia. *Med Care.* 1995;33:771–782.

37. Joranson DE, Gilson AM. State intractable pain policy: current status. *APS Bull.* 1997;7:7–9.

38. Dubois MY. The birth of an ethics charter for pain medicine. *Pain Med.* 2005;6:201–202.

39. Brennan F, Carr DB, Cousins M. Pain management: a fundamental human right. *Anesth Analg.* 2007;105:205–221.

40. Pain IAftSo. Declaration of Montreal: declaration that access to pain management is a fundamental human right. 2010. http://www.iasp-pain.org/Content/NavigationMenu/Advocacy/DeclarationofMontr233al/default.htm.

41. Ballantyne JC, LaForge SL. Opioid dependence and addiction in opioid treated pain patients. *Pain*. 2007;129:235–255.

42. Rubin SB. If we think it's futile, can't we just say no? *HEC Forum*. 2007;19:45–65.

43. Beauchamp TL, Faden RR. The right to health and the right to health care. *J Med Philos*. 1979;4:118–131.

44. Portenoy RK, Foley KM. Chronic use of opioid analgesics in non-malignant pain: report of 38 cases. *Pain*. 1986;25:171–186.

45. Carr DB. *Acute pain management: operative or medical procedures and trauma.* Clinical Practice Guideline. AHCPR Pub No 92-0032. Rockville MD: Agency for Health Care Policy and Research, Public Health Service, US Department of Health and Human Services; 1992.

46. Institute of Medicine of the National Academies Report. *Relieving pain in America: a blueprint for transforming prevention, care, education and research.* Washington, DC: National Academies Press; 2011. http://booksnapedu/openbookphp?record_id=13172&page=53.

    http://www.iom.edu/Reports/2011/Relieving-Pain-in-America-A-Blueprint-for-Transforming-Prevention-Care-Education-Research.aspx

47. Dunn KM, Saunders KW, Rutter CM, et al. Opioid prescriptions for chronic pain and overdose: a cohort study. *Ann Intern Med*. 2010;152:85–92.

48. Saunders KW, Dunn KM, Merrill JO, et al. Relationship of opioid use and dosage levels to fractures in older chronic pain patients. *J Gen Intern Med*. 2010;25:310–315.

49. Gomes T, Mamdani MM, Dhalla IA, Paterson JM, Juurlink DN. Opioid dose and drug-related mortality in patients with nonmalignant pain. *Arch Intern Med*. 2011;171:686–691.

50. Okie S. A flood of opioids, a rising tide of deaths. *N Engl J Med*. 2010;363:1981–1985.

Index

clinical trials for, core
    domains for, for
    treatment efficacy,
    121t
  for complex chronic pain,
    117–22, 118t–122t
  diagnosis importance
    in, 116
  recommendations based
    on, 127
  un-
    ethical issues with,
    126–27
Medicaid, 104
medical comorbidities,
    28–29
medical home, 79
medically unexplained
    symptoms, 2
Medicare, 104
methadone
  coming off of, 89
  drug interactions with,
    92, 94t
  long-term plans for, 98
  in opioid abuse, 24
  in opioid detoxification,
    6
mild traumatic brain injury
    (mTBI), 82
mood disorder, 29
morphine
  for abdominal pain, 3
  drug interactions with, 92
  immediate release, 10
MOR receptor, 46
motor functioning, 107–8
mTBI. See mild traumatic
    brain injury
multidisciplinary
    rehabilitation, 110

N

Narcotics Anonymous, 28
nausea, 98
neck pain, 71
neuropathy
  gabapentin for, 98
  management of, 65–66
  peripheral, HIV related,
    89, 95–96
nociception, 76
nonorganic symptoms, 2
non-steroidal anti-
    inflammatory drug
    (NSAIDs)
  after back surgery, 51
  for cancer pain, 76
  drug interactions with, 92
  for functional pain
    syndrome, 44–45
NSAIDs. See non-steroidal
    anti-inflammatory drug

O

obesity, pain associated
    with, 17
OEF/OIF. See Operation
    Enduring Freedom/
    Operation Iraqi Freedom
Operation Enduring
    Freedom/Operation Iraqi
    Freedom (OEF/OIF), 82
opioid abuse
  during adolescence, 53
  alcoholism with, 20
  buprenorphine role in, 24
  informed consent in,
    22–23
  methadone role in, 24
  obtaining prescriptions in,
    18–19, 136
  red flags for, 17
  requirements for, 90
  with SUD history, 90–91
opioid journey, 4–5
opioid prescribing
    agreement, 23
opioid receptor agonist, 46
Opioid Risk Tool (ORT),
    33t, 124t, 126
opioid screening
  results of, 35
  for risk, 35–36
  role of, 34
  for substance abuse,
    30–31
  tools for, 31–33, 33t
opioid treatment. See also
    chronic opioid treatment
  for abdominal pain, 1–2
  adverse effects from, 124
  aggressive, 83–84
  anger outburst after, 1
  benefits of, 8
  in childhood/adolescence
    case study of, 51–52
    for chronic pain, 52, 61
    considerations for, 51–52
    ethical issues in, 56–57
    long-term consequences
      of, 54
    long-term plan for, 60–61
    monitoring of, 55–56
    recommendations for,
      58–59
    risk of, 59
  comprehensive
    assessment for, 8
  in debilitating pain, 65–69
  denial of, 136
  discontinuing of, 132–33
  ethical issues in, 7–8
  for fibromyalgia, 44
  for functional syndromes,
    47
  goals of, 106

high doses of, 4
  detoxification strategies
    for, 6–9
  immune effects from, 69
  impairment from, 107–9
  injection, 99
  long-term, 72–75
    considerations for, 4–5
    for injured workers
      case, 106
    plans for, 9–10
    safety considerations
      for, 74
    for workers' compensation
      case, 111
  monitoring of
    in childhood/adolescence,
      55–56
    in SUD history, 91
  mood disorders along
    with, 29
  patient perceptions of,
    5–6
  risk assessment for, 35–36
  rotation of, 74
  short-term prescriptions
    in, 19, 136
  in substance abuse
    history, 89–90
    long-term plans for,
      36–37
  in workers' compensation
    case, 109–11
  workplace barriers in,
    for injured workers,
    109–10
ORT. See Opioid Risk Tool
Oswestry Disability Index,
    123t
overdoses
  accidental, history of, 28
  ethical issues in, 35
oxycodone
  APAP/, 15
  doses of, 68
OxyContin®
  costs of, 103
  detoxification from, 127
  use of, 92

P

PADT. See Pain Assessment
    and Documentation Tool
pain. See also specific type i.e.
    abdominal pain
  aggressive treatment
    of, 83
  antidepressant use with,
    66, 94
  anxiety with, 16, 123
  associated obesity, 17
  associated smoking, 16–17
  after back surgery, 27

ch 12   depend on opioids to make life
               tolerable

ch 2 : List of considerations